PSYCHOLOGY RESEARCH PROGRESS

# PSYCHOTHERAPY

## PERSPECTIVES, STRATEGIES AND CHALLENGES

# Psychology Research Progress

Additional books and e-books in this series can be found on Nova's website under the Series tab.

PSYCHOLOGY RESEARCH PROGRESS

# PSYCHOTHERAPY

## PERSPECTIVES, STRATEGIES AND CHALLENGES

HAYLEY BOYD
EDITOR

nova
science publishers
New York

## NOTICE TO THE READER



**Library of Congress Cataloging-in-Publication Data**

ISBN: 978-1-53618-877-6

*Published by Nova Science Publishers, Inc. † New York*

# CONTENTS

# PREFACE

*Psychotherapy: Perspectives, Strategies and Challenges* first discusses the biological components of psychotherapy from the perspective of mechanisms of learning, readaptation, and possible mechanisms of neurogenesis.

Following this, the authors highlight recognizable stages of growing from a novice therapist into a seasoned clinician.

The nuances of the psychotherapeutic process of dynamic psychotherapy are explored, analyzing the role of patients' timing in reaching treatment goals, time as a therapist's tool to provide specific interventions and time as a continuous process of the patient's growth, which does not stop with the end of therapy.

Previous reports showing the ameliorating effects of religious interventions on infectious diseases are reviewed, and possible underlying mechanisms are suggested.

This compilation also reviews the major historical psychoanalytic approaches to psychotherapy that address political issues.

Insights from the discipline of psychology on shame and its relation to aggression are presented in the context of domestic violence and political structures from a critical and feminist standpoint.

The relevance of psychotherapeutic interventions for female breast cancer patients is explored, using accounts that provide crucial information about the psychological experience of the disease.

Additionally, successful psychotherapy for depressive adolescents with suicide attempts is studied in a hospital context.

The effectiveness of psychotherapy and intervention programs conducted with mothers and their children is assessed in an effort to inform families to seek effective treatments and researchers to advance their intervention methods and techniques, which contribute to the healthy development of society.

In closing, it is argued that politically sensitive or socially responsible approaches are bound to play a major role in the renewal of psychotherapy.

Chapter 1 - The analysis of author's psychotherapeutic practice and research in times of the collapse of the USSR and the formation of Russia in comparison with archaic therapeutic practices and basic models of modern psychotherapy led the author to understanding of: the presence in psychotherapy of systemic mechanisms of (a) socio-psychological, (b) psychological (communicative and intrapsychic), (c) (neuro) biological levels; (2) the leading role of mass consciousness, which has a mythological nature and functions, stimulates the development of therapeutic practices that are historically complementary to it and necessitates the adjustment of therapeutic systems to the urgent needs of the "model of the disease and therapy," "model of the problem and its solution" of the mass consciousness; (3) positive acceptance by the patient of the therapeutic system in cases of its complementarity with personal (culturally determined) ideas about illness, problem, with the subsequent inclusion of psychological and biological mechanisms of psychotherapy. The results of research made it possible to formulate the three-component structural-dynamic theory of psychotherapy, describe its components, formulate the concept of a connecting script for psychotherapy, and implement the developed approach in therapeutic practice. Within the framework of the socio-psychological component of psychotherapy, the structure and variants of the mass consciousness dynamics, its "models of the disease and therapy" are described. In the psychological component, the emphasis is on the learning subcomponent and intrapsychic subcomponent are described (the last from the standpoint of the mechanisms of reactivation and the formation of the system of psychological adaptation of the personality, which brings this model closer to the position of positive psychology). The biological component of psychotherapy is discussed from the perspective of mechanisms of learning, readaptation, and possible mechanisms of neurogenesis.

Chapter 2 - The early stages of a career as a psychotherapist can be exhilarating yet challenging. When first learning how to be a psychotherapist, graduate students must juggle a flood of information about psychotherapy while simultaneously forming their own identity as a therapist. The present chapter describes the general stages experienced by novice therapists. 1) Understanding the challenges and fears associated with therapy, 2) Learning the basics of being in the room with a client, 3) Integrating evidence-based practice with common skills, 4) Developing a therapeutic orientation and identity, 5) Continuing the professional evolution. Psychotherapy relies on a supportive bond that has been based in a fiduciary relationship and hope. Over the course of therapy, both therapist and client can learn, change, and grow in important ways. For the novice psychotherapist, the amount of information and knowledge ahead can be simultaneously exciting and daunting. The presented notions are derived through combining the perspectives of a clinician with 30 years of experience in clinical practice with the perspectives of current graduate students at different levels of training. These guidelines are meant to identify and validate the common early stages of becoming a therapist.

Chapter 3 - Dynamic Psychotherapy (DP) emerged with the objective of overcoming the limitations of traditional psychoanalysis, thereby responding to a broader demand of patients who seek help to cope with specific problems in a shorter period of time, and who are unable to accomplish the requirements of a psychoanalytical process. However, as a product of psychoanalysis, the focus of psychodynamic treatment models is the emotional conflicts which are caused by traumatic experiences, not focusing on symptoms alone, but on what they mean. Clinical studies have shown that patients benefit from DP, and that psychoanalysis-based psychotherapies have presented a continuous state of improvement in patients. Nevertheless, these findings are confronted by the fact that many researchers, health professionals and patients discard these psychotherapies because they are long-term treatments, in addition to the qualification and time required for training these therapists. In view of these controversies and convergences, through a vignette-based design, in addition to a literature review, this chapter explores the nuances of the psychotherapeutic process of DP. It analyzes the role of the patient's timing to achieve the treatment goals, time as a therapist's tool to provide specific interventions and time as a continuous process of the patient's growth, which does not stop with the end of therapy. The time of DP has been considered an obstacle to the appropriate investigation of its effectiveness, placing it outside the front-line of treatments for mental disorders. Time is also a reason why patients decline DP, as they often expect to have relatively few therapy sessions, even though their therapists consider the need for longer treatment. DP has traditionally placed emphasis on insight into relationship patterns and the processing of avoided emotions. Since the therapeutic processes involve the delivery of specific emotion-focused interventions tailored to a patient's capacity to process and tolerate feelings, treatments do not have a predetermined duration. This technique aims at helping patients to enhance self-understanding, as well as gain insight into their lives and present-day problems, which may allow them not only to maintain therapeutic improvements but to continue to improve beyond the treatment.

Chapter 4 - Recent decades have seen a tremendous increase in scientific interest regarding the relationship between religion and health. In particular, and in regard to the impact of the Wuhan Coronavirus Disease (COVID-19), the putative effectiveness of religious intervention on infectious diseases has received greater attention worldwide. Indeed, Hummer et al., (2010) analyzed data from a 16-year prospective study of a US representative sample of 20,139 cases, of whom 3,934 were identified as having died. People who attended religious services more than once a week exhibited less than half the risk of death due to infectious disease in the follow-up period compared with those who had never attended. The author's research group has previously reported randomized clinical trials in which a group psychotherapy or prayer based on Happy Science – a religious movement founded by Master Ryuho Okawa in 1986 that has since grown into one of the most influential religious organizations in Japan – doctrine significantly reduces depressive symptoms, which robustly deteriorate a wide range of physical disorders. Moreover, Happy Science has recently published some clinical cases in which Happy Science prayers cured COVID-19. Thus, this article reviews previous reports showing the ameliorating effects of religious interventions on infectious diseases and suggests possible underlying mechanisms.

Chapter 5 - In this article the author reviews major historical psychoanalytic approaches to psychotherapy that had manifestly addressed political issues. In other words, the author wishes to portray the political heritage of psychotherapy, a lost or forgotten one. Contrary to views considering psychotherapy and politics to be antagonistic to one another, these approaches acknowledged the psychopolitical connection. The author believes that this political narrative of psychotherapy is important in the renewal of psychotherapy at present time. The current era is characterized by rapid changes that are bound to affect politics, societies and individuals. These processes of change demand a re-examination of the goals, objectives and methods of psychotherapy. They call for a paradigm shift that may lead to re-inclusion of broad political issues in the psychotherapeutic discourse. The author will argue that in the present historical context, the integration between psychotherapy and politics is necessary.

Chapter 6 - Contextualizing phenomena requires accounting for specifics that evolve over history, such as locally specific morals and values and culture-specific frameworks for sense-making of people`s experiences, as well as political and institutionalized structures. The discipline of psychology usually evokes a division between the individual and her or his sociocultural context as well as between the mind and the body. This double division is rooted in a particular conception of the subject, the self, and emotions, which is prevalent in Western thinking; this conception separates inner experience and outside expression and implies a culture of individuality and interiority (Taylor, 1989; Zaumseil & Schwarz, 2014). By this, the discipline of psychology risks becoming an apolitical approach which helps to reproduce existing power structures by silencing and pathologizing those who are most in need. This article uses insights from the discipline of psychology on shame and its relatedness to aggression and puts them into the contexts of domestic violence and political structures from a critical and feminist standpoint. Shame is used as an analytic tool for the interconnectedness between private experience and a socially structuring moral realm. The shame experience of men as well as that of women in domestic violence contexts is discussed.

Chapter 7 - The purpose of this chapter is to explore the relevance of psychotherapeutic interventions for female breast cancer patients. Little research has been conducted on the individual perception of the disease and its treatments and of the lack of social support among these patients, though in the last forty years, a growing number of breast cancer autobiographies have been published. This chapter is based on thirty such narratives. These accounts provide crucial information about the psychological experience of the disease and suggest that patients tend to harbor intense negative representations of the illness and the treatment protocol as well as acute feelings of isolation, which may have a detrimental impact on their quality of life, affective states, and immune response. Indeed, long-lasting negative emotions and lack of social support have a harmful influence on individuals' quality of life and level of stress, which in turn can have a toxic influence on the person's mental and physical health. Psychotherapy may help to give rise to less threatening representations of breast cancer and treatment and reduce the patients' subjective perception of loneliness. It can also reduce stress and negative mood as well as improve active coping skills and adherence to treatment.

Chapter 8 - Psychotherapy has been shown to be an effective treatment that contributes to individual change and well-being; however, information on how therapeutic change is occurring in depressive adolescents is scarce. Recent studies of psychotherapy show that the study of the process from the therapeutic interaction provides clues to know the subjective dynamism of the patients by focusing on the conversation of the interlocutors. In this sense, the chapter shows a Structure of Therapeutic Conversational Exchanges that allows us to know the internal organization of the dialogues of successful psychotherapies of depressive adolescents with suicide attempts in a hospital context, segmenting the sessions in three main phases and analyzing the time occupied in the production of intra and inter-process exchanges. The exchanges present different movements during the sessions and different moments when they are applied, which are related to the usefulness within the psychotherapy process. This knowledge allows the psychotherapist to know which, when, how to use and manage the Conversational Therapeutic Exchange Structure.

Chapter 9 - Motherhood is a challenging life phase for any woman. Mothers' need for support for childbearing and the risk of psychological disorders increase during this life phase. It is well-known that mothers with mental illnesses usually do not provide sensitive and affectionate parenting to their infants and children. Thereby, children and families may also experience critical negative consequences. For instance, previous studies consistently demonstrated that marital satisfaction is lower among depressed mothers and their husbands. Furthermore, maternal depression is associated with children's insecure attachment and negative representations of self. These negative consequences may intensify when the mothers' psychological disorder goes untreated. Therefore, intervening with these mothers and providing them effective treatment have critical importance for them and their families. Previous literature has displayed various forms of intervention and psychotherapy programs for mothers and their children. These programs included group-based and individual-based psychotherapy for decreasing the level of maternal depression and increasing psychological well-being. Furthermore, several intervention programs were conducted with depressed mothers to promote secure attachment and developmental competence in children. In light of the literature, this chapter aims to review the effectiveness and efficacy of these psychotherapy and intervention programs conducted with mothers and their children. This chapter will inform families to seek effective treatments and researchers to advance their intervention methods and techniques, which contribute to the healthy development of society.

Chapter 10 - This article deals with the era in which we live, an era marked by rapid change on a multitude of planes. The Corona virus pandemic has accelerated and exaggerated the existing trend. The present time is characterized by volatility, uncertainty, complexity and ambiguity (VUCA). These sharp changes necessarily shape or re-construct human subjectivity in ways that bring about further changes both in the individual experience and needs, in interpersonal relations and in social and political trends. In view of these changes, the author believes it to be very apposite to revisit psychotherapy: its theories, tools and activities. The author would like to argue that politically sensitive or socially responsible approaches, that will be described briefly, are bound to play a major role in the renewal of psychotherapy. They may have a unique contribution to the effort of psychotherapists to reconnect to the communities and societies in which they operate, and to become agents of social change.

In: Psychotherapy
Editor: Hayley Boyd
ISBN: 978-1-53618-877-6


*Chapter 1*

# GENERAL THEORETICAL APPROACH TO PSYCHOTHERAPY FROM THE PRACTICAL POSITION: THREE-COMPONENT STRUCTURAL-DYNAMIC THEORY OF PSYCHOTHERAPY

***Rashit Tukaev*[*], *MD***
Department of Psychotherapy and Sexology,
Russian Medical Academy of Continuous Professional Education,
Ministry of Healthcare of the Russian Federation, Moscow, Russia

## ABSTRACT

The analysis of author's psychotherapeutic practice and research in times of the collapse of the USSR and the formation of Russia in comparison with archaic therapeutic practices and basic models of modern psychotherapy led the author to understanding of: the presence in psychotherapy of systemic mechanisms of (a) socio-psychological, (b)

[*] Corresponding Author's E-mail: tukaevrd@gmail.com.

psychological (communicative and intrapsychic), (c) (neuro) biological levels; (2) the leading role of mass consciousness, which has a mythological nature and functions, stimulates the development of therapeutic practices that are historically complementary to it and necessitates the adjustment of therapeutic systems to the urgent needs of the "model of the disease and therapy," "model of the problem and its solution" of the mass consciousness; (3) positive acceptance by the patient of the therapeutic system in cases of its complementarity with personal (culturally determined) ideas about illness, problem, with the subsequent inclusion of psychological and biological mechanisms of psychotherapy.

The results of research made it possible to formulate the three-component structural-dynamic theory of psychotherapy, describe its components, formulate the concept of a connecting script for psychotherapy, and implement the developed approach in therapeutic practice. Within the framework of the socio-psychological component of psychotherapy, the structure and variants of the mass consciousness dynamics, its "models of the disease and therapy" are described. In the psychological component, the emphasis is on the learning subcomponent and intrapsychic subcomponent are described (the last from the standpoint of the mechanisms of reactivation and the formation of the system of psychological adaptation of the personality, which brings this model closer to the position of positive psychology). The biological component of psychotherapy is discussed from the perspective of mechanisms of learning, readaptation, and possible mechanisms of neurogenesis.

**Keywords:** three-component structural-dynamic psychotherapy theory, social-psychologic, psychologic, biologic components, mass consciousness, mechanisms of reactivation and the formation of the system of psychological adaptation of the personality, positive psychology, biologic readaptation mechanisms, neurogenesis.

# 1. Introduction

## 1.1. Practical Prerequisites for the General Theoretical Analysis of Psychotherapy

The author has been involved in clinical psychotherapy of anxiety and affective disorders in Russia since the late 1970s. By the mid-1980s, a distinct mass shift in the reaction of patients to psychotherapy from the initial rational understanding to the irrational-mystical one occurred. Considering the methodological consistency of therapy, the explanation such massive irrational-mystical archaic shift in patients understanding of therapy should have been sought outside the context of the clinic and psychotherapy, in the social processes of the late USSR. This nontrivial hypothesis aroused associatively due to observing the behavior of some initially rational oncological patients, who, at unsuccessful therapeutic situations, interrupted antitumor therapy, switching to archaic therapy of the sorcerer, or healer.

## 1.2. Systemic and Methodological Prerequisites for the General Theoretical Analysis of Psychotherapy

Actual methods of psychotherapy are represented by a wide and sustainable range of practices, which need to be supplemented by a set of methods of traditional therapy. Most of the methods of psychotherapy and traditional practices used by patients have no evidence-based evaluation of the effectiveness. However, it should be assumed that the effectiveness of therapies has no dramatic differences, most likely they are all moderately useful. Such an opinion regarding psychotherapy has been periodically declared in Russia over the past 50 years [1].

The comparable effectiveness of various therapies and practices raises the question of fundamentally similar therapeutic mechanisms that differ from those declared by their adherents.

## 1.3. The Principle of Functional Testing and the Possibility of Its Application in the Study of Psychotherapy.

Modern medicine uses the principle of a functional test, when the dynamics of the investigated indicator for a certain load reveals the analyzed function, mechanism (for example, the ECG test of physical activity). Socio-mediated shift in the perception of therapy can be considered as a very specific functional test that can reveal the general mechanisms of psychotherapy. The noted archaization of the perception of psychotherapy by patients is of particular interest, since it allows to consider the continuum of psychotherapy and healing practices as a single dynamic entity.

### 1.4. Analysis of Psychotherapy in the Inverse Bio-Psycho-Social Paradigm

Psychiatry, close to clinical psychotherapy operates with a bio-psycho-social paradigm [1]. An additional argument for using the paradigm in the analysis of the general mechanisms of psychotherapy is a socially determined shift in the patients' perception of psychotherapy. However, the order of the paradigm components in psychotherapy must be inverted, with its transformation into a socio-psychological-biological paradigm. Therefore, the description of a general theoretical approach to psychotherapy will be based on the systemic analysis of socio-psychological (cultural), psychological, and biological components [2].

## 2. Socio-Psychological Component of Psychotherapy

### 2.1. The Analysis of Psychotherapy Should Take into Account Archaic Forms; Universalism of Ritualization

From the standpoint of psychotherapy, the rites of passage [3] performed during the transition from one phase of the life cycle to another are of the greatest interest. According to A. van Gennep [3], and V. Turner [4], rites of passage have three phases: separation, liminality, and incorporation. In the first separation phase the person is detached from his place in the social group. In the second, liminal phase, the ritual subject left one state but have not yet entered the next passes being devoid of the properties of the past or future state. In the third phase, the ritual subject acquires a new social status and reenter society. V. Turner's term liminoid refers to experiences that have characteristics of liminal experiences but are individualized and do not involve a resolution of a personal crisis. The liminal is temporary part of social or religious ritual, while the liminoid is a break from society. Liminal experiences are rare in industrial societies, being mainly replaced by liminoid experiences.

A comparison of modern psychotherapy methods and rites of passage reveals an amazing formal similarity, based on the deep correspondence of causes, goals, behavioral and communicative means. Modern (primarily group) psychotherapy steadily reproduces various variants of the liminal "communitas," following the meta-goal of the ritual of passage to the next phase of the life cycle for clinical "liminoid" with further transformation into a liminal, with the completion of the third phase of the ritual, integration into society, and recovery. The "communitarian-liminal" form and content of psychotherapy are created unconsciously, being a socially determined and directed, pseudo-spontaneous reproduction of the ritual cycle.

## 2.2. Archaic Forms of Therapy; Commonality

### *2.2.1. Siberian Shamanism and Shamanic Therapy*

Shamanism is a traditional worldview of the indigenous ethnic groups of Siberia [5, 6, 7, 8, 9], which brought to us the archaic religiosity of the Neolithic era. It is based on faith in spirits and the need for special intermediaries between the world of people and the worlds of spirits - shamans, who are elected, trained, endowing with special abilities by spirits.

The shamanistic universe consists of three worlds: the "upper" - skiey, the "middle" - earthly and the "lower" – underground; and man inhabits the "middle" world, and the spirits - "upper" and "lower" ones. The shaman serves the helper for his spirits, guarding his relatives from the troubles with support of spirits.

The shamanic gift is inherited, the transformation into a shaman occurs as a result of the "shamanic disease" [5, 6, 8]. Siberian shamans differ in their supernatural capabilities and functions; great and medium shamans are distinguished [5, 6]. Great shamans possess the entire arsenal of shamanistic practice and can visit all three worlds: the upper, middle and lower. Medium shamans can visit only the middle and lower worlds. Siberian nation of Yakuts divide the shamans into good and evil. Evil shamans - "eduns" are able to bring both benefit and harm, "eat" the "kut" (life force) of a person. According to the beliefs of Altai ethnic groups, a shaman, in addition to good, can be harmful. The strength of the Siberian shaman is determined by the number and list of assistant spirits, their belonging to the upper world, the ruler of which is Ulgen, the middle, earthly world and the lower world, the ruler of which is Erlik. The great shaman has helper spirits from all three worlds. Medium shamans have helper spirits from the middle and lower world.

The most common reason of illness in Siberian shamanism is the abduction of the patient's "kut" (life force) by spirits of the upper or lower world [5, 6, 7, 8]. Less often, an evil spirit infuses a person. The goal of treatment is to return the stolen "kut," or to expel an evil spirit.

The main therapeutic agent is shaman's ritual of "kamlanie" [5, 6, 7, 8, 9]. "Kamlanie" is preceded by divination, during which a causal, "pathogenetic" diagnosis is established. Such a diagnosis includes: determination of the disease typology (mental, somatic); determination of its cause (abduction of "kut" by the spirit, or the introduction of an evil spirit); identification of the "personality" and "domicile" of the spirit that caused the disease. The time of the "kamlanie" is night. Duration - from several hours to several nights. The venue is the patient's home. The patient, his relatives, and fellow villagers are involved in the ritual. During the "kamlanie," shaman, striking a tambourine with a mallet, moves around the patient, dances, declares his own poetic improvisations on traditional themes. The script of "kamlanie" includes gathering the shaman's assistant spirits, diagnostics of the disease, demonstration of the shaman's supernatural abilities, communication with pathogenic spirits aimed at restoring the patient's health, stating the results of ritual, and dismission of the assistant spirits. During the ritual the shaman keeps in touch with the patient and the audience, in order to increase the effectiveness of the "kamlanie," shaman shows them his supernatural abilities (flying, sinking into the ground, bloodlessly inflicting wounds on himself, etc.). It is considered that during "kamlanie" shaman develops controlled trance, while maintaining full contact with the audience.

In case of abduction of the patient's "kut" by spirits, the shaman travels to the upper or lower worlds during the "kamlanie," and if successful, takes away, redeems the "kut" from the abductor, leaving them something in exchange, and returns the "kut" to the patient [5, 6, 7, 8]. The details of the ritual journey are described by the shaman in his chant to the participants, who react vividly to what is happening, often becoming trance witnesses of the shaman's journey and supporting him.

The result of "kamlanie" are distributed in the range from patient's recovery, temporary improvement, to lack of effect and worsening of the condition. The absence of a sufficient effect indicates the need for repeated "kamlanie" by the same shaman, or addressing to another, more experienced and powerful [6, 7].

### *2.2.2. Therapeutic Ritual of Primitive Farmers*

As a therapeutic ritual of primitive farmers, let's analyze the isoma ritual described by V. Turner, which goal is to cure women infertility in Ndembu (Africa) [4].

Infertility is caused by too strong connection of a married woman with the "male side," for which a deceased relative of a woman on the maternal side harms her fertility. He goes to the headwaters of the river flowing near the matrilineal village and utters a spell - "chisaku," which awakens the "shadow" of Isoma, who comes to a victim in a dream in the guise of the spirit of Mwenga, whose clothes ropes block female fertility.

Ritual divination preceded the treatment. The isoma treatment consists in: finding by the healers the burrows of a rat or anteater near the river where the isoma spell was pronounced; instillation of "medicines," with the utterance of a spell; digging of "hot" and "cold" sacred pits connected by a tunnel, clearing the ritual space around; giving a woman a white chicken - a symbol of fertility and health, wetting spouses with "medicines"; passage of spouses from the "hot" pit to the "cold" pit through the tunnel; drinking by participants of beer, sprinkling of spouses with "medicines"; decapitation of the red rooster - the destruction of "chisaku"; re-sprinkling of spouses with "medicines"; singing by adherents of ritual songs of life passage.

### *2.2.3. Ritual Therapy of Russian Peasants in 17-19 Centuries*

The worldview of the Russian peasantry of that historical period has a religious and magical basis [10, 11]. The Orthodox Christian shell is saturated with an essentially pagan, ceremonial-magical content.

The three-part World consists of Heaven with Paradise, Earth, underground Hell. The world is ruled by the Lord God, the Lord of Hell is the Devil, Man lives on Earth. The world is full of supernatural forces of Good and Evil, good and evil spirits associated with the forces of Paradise and Hell. In addition, the Earth is inhabited by pagan spirits of nature, polarized between Good and Evil, sometimes ambivalent. At the same time, earthly life presents the subject of the natural factors influences.

A person is able to directly appeal to God, angels, saints, however, without priests, part of the necessary rites is impossible. A person can directly appeal to the forces of Evil, but this interaction is improved due to intermediaries - witches and sorcerers. Influence on supernatural powers is carried out in the form of prayers, verbal ritual magic, subject-ritual magic.

The causes of diseases are divided into natural and supernatural [11]. Natural causes of illness: colds, physical overstrain. A cold is defined as a disease in which a general feeling of cold occurs, it includes: rheumatism, fever, typhoid, erysipelas, pulmonary diseases. Physical overstrain generates such diseases as "tear," "navel disruption" (diseases of the musculoskeletal system, gastrointestinal disorders).

The pathological process develops from outside to inside, if it penetrates deeply, a person will die. Therefore, it is necessary to move the disease out. Dissemination to inside occurs with blood flow, therefore, "bad" and "stagnant" blood must be "released."

Supernatural causes of disease are more numerous. Diseases can be filled with God, as a punishment for sins, sometimes as a teaching. Fighting such diseases is useless. More often, diseases are sent by pagan spirits (leshiy, kikimora), or by the Devil. The Devil is the father of all diseases, diseases sent by the Devil are the most difficult to treat. Diseases can be caused by people mediating the influence of evil spirits (spoilage, evil eye, fright) [10, 11, 12, 13]. Evil eye can send by healers, sorcerers, witches. Evil eye can be temporary, or permanent, until death. The incurable Evil eye can be removed by the sorcerer who sent it, or by a stronger sorcerer.

A wide range of people is involved in magical, spell-ritual therapy: sorcerers, and witches, medicine-men, holy elders, clergymen [10, 11, 13, 14]. Sorcerers and witches are intermediaries between man and evil spirits, the Devil. The basis of the magical influence of the sorcerer, the witch on man and nature - rituals and spells. Sorcerers and witches are capable send evil eye, triggering disease on people and livestock, causing adverse weather events. At the same time, they can treat many diseases, especially those sent by them, however, this treatment, being effective, uses devilish power.

The medicine-men mainly serve as intermediaries between man and God, although in some cases they cooperate with evil spirits. Through spells and prayers, they have the ability to heal people and animals, although they can send diseases.

The religious and social functions of the clergyman are extremely wide, include healing, based on exorcism. [11]. The holy elders, who have a constant connection with the divine world, are able to have a direct and indirect (through prayers, rituals) harmonizing and healing effects on people. In the treatment by witchcraft and prayer, the therapeutic ritual uses spells - special formulaic texts.

Spells are genetically related to the myths that generated them and are abbreviations, applications of myths. The general scheme of the spell and the myth: "action - change (new state) - action, taking into account the achieved new state - the desired result. The spell formula has a complex semantic structure, is saturated with mythological and ritual symbolism, but is opaque, hidden from both the healer and the patient [15]. For the healer and the patient, the spell presents the mandatory formula that includes necessary set of sacred magic symbols, listing them in the prescribed sequence provides the desired result.

If treatment is unsuccessful, its intensity should be increased. If the treatment with an appeal to God does not help, it is radicalized by an appeal to the Devil, an evil spirit (through an intermediary sorcerer).

### *2.2.4. Magical Thinking. The Position of J. G. Frazer*

J. G. Frazer [16] singled out two laws on which magical thinking is based: the law of similarity, according to which the effect resembles its cause; the law of, according to which objects that have touched once, continue to interact after the end of the contact. Magical practice implements the law of similarity in homeopathic and the law of contagion - in contagious magic.

### *2.2.5. The Patterns of Historical Dynamics of Therapeutic Rituals*

The comparison of various types of archaic therapy, including shaman's "kamlanie," the therapeutic ritual of primitive farmers, and healers spell therapy indicates that the complications of social life and labor activity leads to a change in the form and symbolism of therapeutic rituals.

The change in therapeutic rituals is manifested in: 1) a change in the method of magical action; 2) the degree of participation of a social group in the ritual; 3) changing the ritual procedure; 4) changing the symbolism of the ritual.

For each historical era, magical action presents an analogue of life-sustaining activity. For collector and hunter societies, the most universal way of activity was to move in space, because only it could lead to the goal of obtaining food and maintaining life. In a primitive agricultural society, life became hand-made, because, first of all, manual labor, i.e., manual-objective manipulations, provided life. With the advent of complex, developed social institutions (of state), the oral and written speech of the rulers, the carrier of verbal-symbolic action, began to play a decisive role in people's life.

The magical action in its historical development passed through similar stages, manifesting in: the magic of movement in space (flight of a shaman to the upper and lower worlds); manual-subject magic (rites of primitive farmers); verbal-symbolic magic (spells). Of course, this distinction is relative, since any magic is symbolic and already in the magical actions of the shaman all three types of magic are present as elements, but, nevertheless, their predominant representation in each case is different.

The degree of participation of social group in the transition from shamanistic and agricultural therapeutic rituals to spells decreases, the magical effect from public becomes more and more individual.

On the path to the historical transformation of the magical therapeutic ritual, especially in the transition to spells, there occurs a significant reduction, simplification of the ritual, reducing it mainly to a rather short verbal formula.

The symbolism of therapeutic rituals during their historical transformation also changes significantly.

1. The semantic content of the symbols of the ritual with the historical simplification of the form becomes more ambiguous, due to the absorption of the main symbolic constructs of previous rituals.
2. Ritual symbolism develops from primary, concrete-subject to secondary, universal, abstract-symbolic, replacing the multiple primary symbols of a given method of magical action with a basic symbol expressing the essence of such magical actions.
3. In the process of historical development, ritual symbolism becomes increasingly incomprehensible to the performer and user of the ritual, which is most typical for spells.
4. The growing popularity of healing in society will probably indicate a regressive archaization of mass consciousness.

## 2.3. Comparative Analysis of Some Modern Psychotherapeutic Systems

Modern psychotherapy is represented by a great number of methods, grouped into three main approaches: psychodynamic, cognitive-behavioral, existential; the aggregate analysis of which in a separate chapter is impossible. Therefore, in an extremely formal way, the iconic methods of Western psychotherapy (classical psychoanalysis, object relations therapy, cognitive therapy) and the Russian method of personality-oriented psychotherapy will be analyzed.

### *2.3.1. Psychoanalytic Approach*

#### 2.3.1.1. Classical Psychoanalysis of Z. Freud

According to the mature Freud [17-23], the model of personality is represented by three components: Id (unconsciously biological, reduced to energy of libido), Ego (core of personality, constantly matching the requirements of Reality, Id and Super-ego), Super-ego (social, formed in childhood on the basis of the Oedipus or Electra complexes and subsequently unchanged). The Id presents main motivational sphere, the Ego is its interpreter. Sexual libidinal and genital functions are separated. The libido in its development goes through the oral, anal-sadistic, genital stages, forming the Oedipus complex (the period of the son's heightened attachment to the mother, with hostility to the father), or the Electra complex (the period of the daughter's heightened attachment to the father, with the hostility to the mother). In addition to the libido, the ID includes the death instinct (Thanatos) - the desire for self-destruction, expressed in acts of hetero - and auto-aggression, the existence of the individual is a compromise between them. Personal anxiety is caused by pressure on the Ego of Reality, Id, Super-ego. The Ego is saved from the emerging stress through the mechanisms of psychological defenses.

Neurosis is the consequence of an unsuccessful defense process, the result of a weakening of the Ego's strength due to the pressure of the Id and the dissipation of energy to counter this pressure, or neurosis is a conflict between the Super-ego and the Ego. The roots of neurosis are in early childhood. The goal of psychoanalytic therapy is to resolve the neurotic conflict, i.e., strengthening the Ego, its independence from the Super-ego, changing its organization and expanding the field of perception with the possibility of a more complete mastering of Id.

Classical psychoanalysis includes the steps of: material production, analysis, working alliance. The main methods of material production are: free associations, transfer, resistance. Analysis of the patient's material includes: confrontation, clarification, interpretation, study. The working alliance implies a rational relationship between the patient and the analyst, which makes the process of psychotherapy goal-oriented. Essential methods of psychoanalysis are also: the "rule of abstinence" and "the analyst as a mirror." The "rule of abstinence" is based on the patient's suffering in the process of analysis, and the suffering must reach such an extent that it becomes effective in work. The term "analyst as a mirror" implies a behavior in which the analyst remains "dark," impenetrable to the patient, but not cold-heartless.

#### 2.3.1.2. Object Relations Therapy

The development of psychoanalytic theory led to the formation of the theory and therapy of object relations [24, 25, 26], the distinguishing feature of which is the shift in emphasis from instinct to relationship. In order to understand an individual, it is necessary to understand his self-representations, ideas about objects and object relations. This inevitably leads to an understanding of the individual's early relationships with the person who provided the main care for him. The individual, on the basis of these early experiences, forms patterns, stereotypes that subsequently affect perception, thinking, feeling and establishing relationships. Disturbance of the object relations of the developing Ego will determine the roots of all psychopathological conditions [27]. The main problem is the defect of the environment or the lack of sufficiently good maternal care. Therapy of object relations is built as a replacement therapy. It involves replacing bad objects with good ones. Its objective is to give the patient relationships in which the “frozen parts” of his Self would have gained the opportunity to develop, in which the impaired development would be restored, making it possible for the patient to reborn. First of all, intervention requires a good relationship between the psychoanalyst and the patient. Therapy uses “good” personal relationships to eliminate the harm from early “bad” relationships [250]. Regression and transference analysis are important components of the intervention. The psychoanalyst, with some delay, corrects that which initially failed to make the “insufficiently good” mother [25].

### *2.3.2. Cognitive Therapy*

A. Beck’s cognitive therapy [28, 29, 30] is based on the idea that the words and thoughts of people are of great importance. Along with conscious thoughts, unconscious, automatic thoughts are arising. Automatic thoughts consist of ideas that other people consider irrational (however, they seem quite reasonable to the person), as well as the rules and laws, according to which the person judges his actions and plans strategies for behavior. These rules can lead to non-adaptive actions. People react to events interpreting them depending on their influence on individual’s Self.

The result of the interpretations are various emotions. Interpretations containing a distortion of reality lead to emotional disorders, which in reality are disorders of thinking. Disturbed thinking includes personalization of events, polarizing thoughts, applying rules in an unconditional, absolutist manner.

Cognitive therapy aims to weaken emotional disorders by correcting false interpretations of reality and erroneous judgments. The therapist and patient establish a cooperative relationship with attention to solving problems, rather than correcting personal defects.

A. Beck with colleagues and followers have developed effective approaches to the treatment of depressive, anxiety, phobic, personality disorders.

### *2.3.3. Russian Methods of Personal-Oriented Psychotherapy*

The founder of personality-oriented psychotherapy, V. M. Myasishchev [31], defined personality as a social formation, a system of relations with people, forming in ontogenesis, in the given socio-historical and economic, everyday conditions. Relations is a conscious, empirical-selective psychological connection of a person with various aspects of life, expressed in his actions, reactions, experiences. Relationships are characterized by: level of activity, the interrelation of rational and irrational, conscious and unconscious, stability and instability. From the standpoint of the psychology of relations, neurosis is a psychogenic, caused by conflicts neuropsychic disorder based on the disturbance of personality-significant relationships. The goals and objectives of personality-oriented therapy [1, 31, 32] are: the study of personality, the specifics of the patient's relationship system; the study of etiopathogenetic mechanisms of the onset and preservation of a neurotic state; the achievement of patient awareness of the cause-effect relationship of a relationship system and disease; help the patient in a reasonable resolution of a situation; change in the patient's relationship with behavior correction. The applied methods of psychotherapy are individual and group, using the mechanisms of group dynamics.

### *2.3.4. Comparison of the Described Methods of Psychotherapy*

Preceding analysis of the methods of archaic magical therapy revealed several important points. Let us emphasize two: 1) the correlation of magical action with the social life and ideology of the corresponding era, or rather, the conditionality of the form and context of magical action and therapy by actual social life and ideology; 2) at the next step in the development magic ritual introjects and retains in a symbolic form, the previous magical action. The question arises, are these points of magical therapeutic rituals development persist in the field of modern psychotherapy? The answer to both points is positive.

Thus, the early basic psychoanalytic construct of the irrationality of mental life, according to E. Fromm [33-36], is secondary and reflects the idea of irrationality that prevailed in the West on the eve of World War I. It also seems logical that therapy of object relations and cognitive therapy, which emerged in the era of the successful post-war reconstruction of Western Europe in the 1950s on the basis of the Marshall Plan, implement therapy as a positive, rational reconstruction of the psyche, distorted in the early period of development, based on corrective cooperation. Russian personality-reconstructive therapy in its interpretation of personality is based on the definition of K. Marx (a person is a set of social relations) [37], which became part of the ideology of the Soviet period.

It should be recognized that orthodox psychoanalysis had a profound impact not only on the development of all subsequent psychotherapy, introducing its own positive or negative introjects (including the examples given earlier), but also became a component of Western culture and mass consciousness. In general, psychotherapy, as well as magic therapy, appears to be a secondary phenomenon in relation to social life, worldview, mass consciousness, historically changing after the changes in the latter. The relative simplicity and integrity of social life, worldview, mass consciousness of the times of magic therapy generate its universalism, the undifferentiated set of concepts and means, fully incorporated into social life and culture. And, on the contrary, the complexity and differentiation of modern social life, worldview, and mass consciousness give rise to sufficient isolation, specificity of concepts and means of psychotherapy, creating the impression of its self-sufficiency.

Modern psychotherapies are dualistic, have proclaimed, conscious theoretical basis and set of techniques, developing in response to an actual, but less conscious social, cultural requests.

## 2.4. Mass Consciousness, "Model of Disease and Therapy"

So, the analysis showed that psychotherapy in its historical development follows social life, changes in mass consciousness [2].

### *2.4.1. "Model of Disease and Therapy"*

Seeking medical help for various diseases, the patient already has initial common ideas about the presence and characteristics of diseases, about how he will be provided with medical care on the base of his own experience of diseases and certain general cultural knowledge and norms. In the most general form, the provision of medical care is understood as step-by-step sequential: "examination," "diagnostics," "treatment." Certain knowledge about diseases, their severity, outcomes, sequence, types and forms of medical care is acquired by a person both directly, through the experience of diseases and their treatment, and indirectly, through the experience of other people's illnesses, accumulated, transformed from the surrounding socio-cultural environment.

The author considers that people's ideas about the causes of diseases and their treatment are not accidental and form a complex system that can be defined as a "Model of Illness and Therapy" (MDT), the repository of which is the mass, everyday consciousness [2, 38, 39].

"Model of a disease" is a set of the most generalized, middling knowledge, ideas, opinions of people about diseases, their types, causes, treatment characteristics, and outcomes. The "Model of the Disease" is inextricably linked with the "Model of Therapy" - a set of generalized, middling knowledge, judgments, opinions and ideas about methods of treatment, their effectiveness, mechanisms.

The MDT - the medical component of mass consciousness is practically unexplored, while its study is of considerable interest not only for psychotherapy, but, undoubtedly, for therapeutic disciplines in general. The MDT of mass consciousness is a component of the "Model of the World" of mass consciousness, which represents a systematic description of the world and man. From the standpoint of psychotherapy, one should single out in the "Model of the World" of mass consciousness such a component as "Model of the problem and its solution."

In typical cases, in the process of treatment of diseases, medical measures do not go beyond the traditional, stage-by-stage "Examination," "Diagnostics" and "Therapy" of "Model of Disease and Therapy," therefore, the patient's acceptance of the treatment is in line with his expectations. Modern methods of psychotherapy are probably the least traditional from the standpoint of the actual MDT, and therefore must use the means to maintain social attractiveness and effectiveness.

Traditional, generally accepted methods of psychotherapy (psychoanalysis, cognitive-behavioral therapy) have already been assimilated by the MDT of the Western mass consciousness. New psychotherapy methods that have developed their own techniques are not included in the MDT of mass consciousness and need to be explained to patients. Therefore, all relatively new methods of psychotherapy at the beginning of work with a patient include the presentation of a connecting script of subsequent therapy, with description of goals, objectives, normative roles, procedures, and expected results. Such a connecting script can be presented in a structured form at the beginning of therapy, or it will be clarified during therapy, at its beginning.

Thus, the development of modern psychotherapy, as well as the historical dynamics of archaic forms of therapy, are determined by uniform laws.

1. The conceptual foundations of the current psychotherapeutic system are in accordance with its contemporary MDT of mass consciousness. The relative discrepancies between the psychotherapeutic system and the model of illness and therapy are overcome with the help of a connecting script that allows to overcome the differences existing between them.
2. The development of psychotherapy and the dynamics of the MDT represent a single dialectical process with a system of direct and feedback connections, in which the historical, socially determined dynamics of mass consciousness and the MDT determine the development of psychotherapy, while the theoretical foundations of the psychotherapeutic system, which formulated and proposed the solution of urgent existential problems are included in the social ideology, penetrating into the mass consciousness.
3. The process of historical development of the mass consciousness MDT and psychotherapy has a qualitative integrity, continuity and

is based on the accumulation, specific "conservation" of the previous traditional social models of decision. This is illustrated by the pseudo-spontaneous restoration of the semantic structure of the rites of passage in modern group psychotherapy, using the ritual cliché, crystallized millennia earlier for solving of similar problems.

## 2.5. Structure, Variants of Dynamics and Historical Development of the Model of Disease and Therapy of Mass Consciousness

As noted in the chapter introduction, the author became interested in the nature of psychotherapy after the archaization of his patients' attitudes towards his psychotherapy. For explanation, the hypothesis of archaization of mass consciousness was proposed as a result of a social deadlock developing in the life of the late USSR on the eve of the 1990s [2, 38, 39]. In those years, there happened a boom in extrasensory healing, newspapers talked about different magicians, A. Kashpirovsky, A. Chumak, D. Davitashvili consistently became TV stars, replacing each other. The author, observing extremely curious events, became interested in the possibility of an experimental study of the initial representations of people about diseases and their therapy (MDT) and the search for signs of archaization of these representations in: 1) an experimentally created deadlock situation; 2) persons involved in training in psychic therapy. Such a study was implemented, its results are described below.

### *2.5.1. The Experimental Method "Model of Disease and Therapy"*

The method "Model of Disease and Therapy" was developed by the author for study of human representations about the effectiveness of various types of diseases treatment. The method is based on the principle of rank grid method of D. Bannister [40]. The rank grid presents a matrix filled in during the survey, which includes elements and constructs. Elements are groups of objects from a specific area that are reasonably related. Constructs are bipolar-scaled features that relate to the area characterized by the elements.

Our test uses the possible outcomes of different treatments as 7 elements [2, 39]:

- Element 1. Treatment is useless.
- Element 2. Treatment brings minor temporary improvement.
- Element 3. Treatment brings clear temporary relief.
- Element 4. Treatment leads to gradual significant improvement in the condition.
- Element 5. Treatment leads to gradual recovery.
- Element 6. Treatment leads to rapid full recovery.
- Element 7. Treatment leads to sudden full recovery.

The constructs are described in the language of the average patient. The 14 constructs describe various types of treatment, from traditional magical, attributed to "traditional medicine," to conventional in medicine, and, finally, high-tech:

- Construct 1. Treatment of a person with extraordinary abilities in recognizing and treating diseases, for example, a psychic who has the ability to sense the biofield and use it for therapeutic effects.
- Construct 2. Treatment by an experienced chiropractor.
- Construct 3. Treatment by an experienced healer, treating with special herbs, potions, spells.
- Construct 4. Treatment by a qualified psychotherapist (hypnosis, autogenous training, group psychotherapy, other types of psychotherapy).
- Construct 5. Treatment with medical massage.
- Construct 6. Treatment by a qualified acupuncturist.
- Construct 7. Treatment with medical tinctures, potions, drops, prescribed by a doctor.
- Construct 8. Treatment with pills, prescribed by a doctor.

- Construct 9. Treatment with subcutaneous, intramuscular injections, prescribed by a doctor.
- Construct 10. Treatment with intravenous injections, droppers, prescribed by a doctor.
- Construct 11. Treatment with electrical procedures (like electrophoresis).
- Construct 12. Treatment with balneological agents (baths, mud).
- Construct 13. Treatment by surgical means (operations).
- Construct 14. Treatment with modern technical means (laser, radioactive substances, ultrasound and others).

The procedure of psychological research was as follows. All 7 elements and the 1st construct are presented to the Subject. The subject is asked to indicate the element (treatment result) that most fully characterizes the given construct (type of therapy). The indicated element is removed from, and the subject is again asked to indicate the element (treatment result), most completely, of the remaining, characterizing this construct (type of therapy). The procedure is repeated until the last element remains. When all 7 elements are ranked by 1 construct, construct 2 is presented, its ranking procedure is carried out, similar to the ranking of construct 1. After the ranking is completed by 7 elements of all 14 constructs, a 7 × 14 element ranking matrix is obtained.

Modern man has not only a general representation about medicine, but also distinguishes between its individual areas: diseases in general, therapy, surgery, oncology, infections, etc. Therefore, the method provides, on the base of goal setting of a concrete study, the assessment of representations about a specific field of medicine by highlighting the testing theme that is demonstrated to the subject in the testing cycle, when working with constructs and elements.

The ranking results are entered in the protocol form (with a 7 × 14 matrix). Constructs are columns, elements are rows. To assess the group results, the indicator of the sum of the scores of the relationships for each construct of the individual matrix, proposed by D. Bannister, was used; it characterizes the general variance explained by this construct. For each pair of rankings of individual matrix, using Spearman's rank correlation coefficient, the scores of the relationship (p2 × 100) are calculated, which are then summed up for each construct without taking into account the sign. The sums of the scores of the relationships of the 14 constructs of the tested selected groups were subsequently subjected to the standard procedure of factor analysis by the method of principal components).

### *2.5.2. Experimental Psychological Study of the Structure and Dynamics of the Model of Disease and Therapy*

#### 2.5.2.1. The Objectives of the Study

1. Revealing the archaization of representations about diseases and their therapy in adult subjects in a situation of an experimental impasse;
2. Comparison of the archaization of representations about diseases and their therapy in adult subjects in an experimental situation with the archaization of representations of diseases and their therapy in adult subjects who reacted to a social dead-end situation.

To achieve the first goal in 1989 (3 years after the Chernobyl disaster), 60 workers of the plant in the city of Mozyr (70 km from the Chernobyl nuclear power plant), during a preventive medical examination, on condition of voluntary informed consent, twice, with an interval of 5 minutes, were tested according to the MDT method; the theme of the first study is "Diseases in general," the theme of the second study is "Diseases caused by radiation." The author suggested that the second theme would actualize the experimental impasse and cause archaization of representations about diseases and their therapy.

To achieve the second goal in 1990, during the period of active disintegration processes in the USSR, accompanied by a sharp increase in interest in psychic healing, 106 students at the "school of psychics" in the Ufa city, during a medical examination, on the basis of voluntary informed consent, a single test was carried out on the MDT method; research theme -

"Diseases in general." The author suggested that persons studying extrasensory healing during the collapse of the USSR had already, and most sharply, reacted to the social dead-end situation and would initially demonstrate archaization of representations about diseases and their therapy.

The study design for both groups included MDT testing method: for the Mozyr group - twice, with an interval of 5 minutes, using the first theme "Diseases in General" and the second - "Diseases caused by radiation"; for Ufa group once using the theme "Diseases in General."

#### 2.5.2.2. Materials and Methods

The Mozyr group consisted of 60 subjects, 37 women (62%), 23 men (38%), aged from 27 to 52 years (average age - 38.5 ± 5.2 years). The Ufa group included 106 subjects, 68 women (64%), 38 men (36%), aged from 22 to 55 years (average age - 43.4 ± 6.7 years).

In the study, according to the design, the MDT method was applied, the themes "Diseases in General" and "Diseases caused by radiation" were used.

Statistical processing was performed using the Statistica 6.0 software. The sums of the scores of the relationships of Mozyr and Ufa groups were applied in factor analysis by the method of principal components.

#### 2.5.2.3. Results of Research

The results of factor analysis of the MDT testing for the Mozyr group data are presented in Tables 1, 2, and the analogous data for Ufa group -in Table 3. The names of the factors were given on the basis of a generalized interpretation of the totality of the variables included in them. The definition "External" methods of therapy characterize the methods of therapy that act through the surface of the body, the skin. The definition "Internal" therapy refers to therapies that act primarily through the mouth or ears.

**Table 1. Mozyr Factor matrix of scores for the relationship of assessing the effectiveness of therapy for "diseases in general"**

| Factor | Factor name | Variables and their meanings |
|---|---|---|
| F1 | Conservative therapy | Tablets (0.83), Injections (0.81), Electrotherapy (0.76), Droppers (0.76), Tinctures (0.68), 0, Balneotherapy (0.67), Modern technical therapy (0.57) |
| F2 | Radical therapy | Surgery (0.79), Modern technical therapy (0.57) |
| F3 | Traditional therapy | Acupuncture (0.79), Massage (0.56) |
| F4 | Methods of therapeutic mental influence | Psychotherapy (0.87), Psychic Treatment (0.59) |
| F5 | - | Chiropractor Treatment (0,94) |
| F6 | - | Healer's Treatment (0.91) |
| Number of subjects | 60 | |
| Dispersion | 86% | |

**Table 2. Mozyr Factor matrix of scores for the relationship of evaluating the effectiveness of therapy for diseases associated with radiation**

| Factor | Factor name | Variables and their meanings |
|---|---|---|
| F1 | "External" Methods of Therapy | Acupuncture (0.91), Massage (0.69), Electrotherapy (0.61), Balneotherapy (0.60), Modern technical therapy (0.56), Chiropractor treatment (0.94) |
| F2 | "Internal" Methods of Therapy | Droppers (0.79), Psychotherapy (0.71), Injection (0.71), Tablets (0.71), |
| F3 | | Tinctures (0.87) |
| F4 | | Healer's Therapy (0.83) |
| F5 | | Psychic Treatment (0.92) |
| F6 | | Surgery (0.91) |
| Number of subjects | 60 | |
| Dispersion | 88% | |

**Table 3. Ufa Factor matrix of scores for the relationship of assessing the effectiveness of therapy for "disease in general" by students of the school of psychics**

| Factor | Factor name | Variables and their meanings |
|---|---|---|
| F1 | Magic therapy | Healer's treatment (0.76), Acupuncture (0.72), Psychotherapy (0.68), Chiropractor treatment (0.63) |
| F2 | "Internal" Methods of Therapy | Injections (0.78), Droppers (0.74), Tinctures (0.59), Tablets (0.57) |
| F3 | "External" Methods of Therapy | Electrotherapy (0.82), Balneotherapy (0.75), Massage (0.62) |
| F4 | - | Modern technical therapy (0,73) |
| F5 | - | Surgery (0,78) |
| F6 | | Psychic Treatment (0,83) |
| Number of subjects | 106 | |
| Dispersion | 81% | |

The factor matrix for evaluating the therapy of "disease in general" is presented in Table 1 and consists of 6 factors (the variables of which are given in decreasing order of significance). The first factor – "Conservative Therapeutic Methods of Treatment includes: treatment with pills, injections, electrotherapy, treatment with droppers, tinctures, balneological treatment, treatment with modern technical means. The second factor - radical therapeutic methods of treatment includes: surgical treatment, treatment with modern technical means. The third factor is formed by traditional medical methods of manual treatment: acupuncture, medical massage. The fourth factor presents the methods of therapeutic mental influence: psychotherapy, psychic treatment. Factors five and six include single variables: treatment of the chiropractor and the healer.

The factor matrix for evaluating the therapy of "radiation-related diseases" by the Mozyr group is shown in Table 2 and consists of 6 factors (the variables of which are given in decreasing order of significance).

The first factor of "External" methods of therapy includes: acupuncture, massage, electrotherapy, balneological treatment, treatment with modern technical means, chiropractor treatment. The second factor of "Internal" methods of therapy includes: treatment with droppers, psychotherapy, treatment with injections, pills. Factors from the third to the sixth include, single variables: treatment with tinctures, treatment of a medicine man, treatment of a psychic, surgical treatment.

The survey of students of the school of psychics was carried out during the boom of psychic healing in the spring of 1991. The factor matrix of scores for the relationship of evaluating the effectiveness of therapy of the "disease in general" by the students of the school of psychics is given in Table 3 and consists of 6 factors (the variables are arranged in decreasing order of significance).

The first factor of Traditional magical methods of treatment includes: Healer's treatment, Acupuncture, Psychotherapy, Chiropractor treatment. The second factor of medical methods of "internal" treatment includes: treatment with injections, droppers, tinctures, tablets. The third factor presents medical methods of "external" treatment, including: electrotherapy, balneotherapy, medical massage. Factors from three to six include single variables: Modern technical therapy, Surgery, Psychic treatment.

#### 2.5.2.4. Modern and Archaic Models of Disease and Therapy on the Base of Test Results: Discussion

The first Mozyr factor matrix, which includes the subject's assessments of supposed effectiveness of the treatment of "disease in general," characterizes the MDT, which classifies various methods of therapy according to their presence in real life and adequately evaluates their significance: the dominance of conservative therapeutic methods, the important role of surgery and other modern technical methods, sufficient relevance, the proximity of traditional medical methods of acupuncture and massage. Psychotherapy, extrasensory therapy, chiropractor treatment, a healer, are combined, which justifiably gives grounds to define them as "Methods of therapeutic mental influence."

The second Mozyr factor matrix, obtained during the examination of the same subjects, practically at the same time, but representing an extremely significant, threatening for those living in the Chernobyl accident zone, an assessment of the effectiveness of treatment of "diseases caused by radiation" (requiring essentially the same structure of medical care), is qualitatively different. The subjects unexpectedly divided the therapy methods based on the bipolar trait "external" - "internal." Moderately significant in the previous "model of disease and therapy" and the most ancient of all traditional medical methods of treatment - acupuncture and massage, are assessed in the second survey as the most significant, leading the first factor of this matrix, which also includes the treatment of the chiropractor, while the indicator of surgical treatment, which headed the second factor of the first matrix, becomes the least significant. The MDT, actualized by the conditions of an experimental deadlock, loses its connection with the modern therapeutic reality and a different, archaic structure and content clearly appears in it.

The factorial matrix for evaluating the effectiveness of treatment of "diseases in general" by students of the school of psychics is close to the Mozyr matrix of "diseases caused by radiation" and is also distant from modern therapeutic reality, since it highlights "internal" and "external" methods of treatment, reduces the importance of surgery. But, in contrast to the compared one, in this model the most significant are traditional methods of treatment (acupuncture, psychotherapy, chiropractor treatment), which acquire a magical coloring due to the leadership of the healer therapy in this group. It is interesting that the indicator of psychic treatment is highlighted by the students in the last factor of the matrix, and, having a high significance (0.83), is separated from all other methods of treatment. This is due to the fact that extrasensory perception was understood by teachers and students as a fundamentally new, scientific, developing, if not refuting modern medicine, method of diagnosis and therapy. The last factorial matrix reflects the most archaized MDT, which is acquiring a frankly magical coloring.

The division of therapy methods into "external" and "internal," revealed in two archaized factor matrices, is, in our opinion, related to archaic MDT. This circumstance prompts the search for similar classifications of therapeutic techniques in traditional systems of therapy with archaic roots, which inevitably preserved, systematized, developed the provisions of the MDT of mass consciousness that corresponded to the period of their formation.

The most developed traditional systems of therapy are the Chinese, Tibetan and Arab ones. Indeed, these systems have developed fundamental concepts of the "external" and "internal" causes of diseases (in line with the ideas of the connection between the Universe and humans) about the clinic, diagnostics, "external" and "internal" treatment.

In classical Chinese medicine, the categories of "internal" and "external" are codified in the concept of yin - yang (yin corresponds to "internal" and yang to "external") [41], they develop in the concept of the cycle of interconversions of Wu Xing, are included in dialectics " I Ching "(" Books of Changes ") [42] and are most consistently implemented in the theory and practice of pulse diagnostics and zhen - chiu therapy [41].

In the Tibetan medical science Zhud-shi, the system of medicine is represented in the form of nine trees growing from three roots [43]. Four trees grow from the third root, the first symbolizes food and drink, the second - the way of life, the third - medicinal substances ("Man") taken internally, the fourth symbolizes external methods of treatment, including surgery ("Shad").

Avicenna, who reflected in the "Canon of Medicine" [44] the achievements of Arab-Persian medicine at the end of the first millennium, subdivided, referring to Galen, all diseases into external and internal, distinguishing three types of therapy: regimen and nutrition; drug administration ("internal" treatment); hand action ("external" treatment).

Thus, the similarity of two factorial matrices showing archaized MDT is a natural phenomenon based on the actualization of previous "models" accumulated, "conserved" in the mass consciousness in the course of the historical development of MDT. It should be noted that the first archaic factor matrix was obtained during a psychological examination and reflects the experimentally determined, individual regressive dynamics of the previously relevant modern MBT when the subject is placed in a situation that is insoluble from the standpoint of this model. The factor matrix of the students of the school of psychics revealed the "background," actual at the time of the survey, the most archaic of the three MDT's, obtained for persons who have a short interest in psychic therapy (4-6 months) and, for the most part, who had not previously thought about it. It can be reasonably assumed that this archaized MDT is a consequence of the regressive dynamics of the modern model under the influence of not an individual, but a socially conditioned cause, which in its meaning is close to an insoluble disease situation.

If we assume that the first, background factorial matrix of the Mozyr series reflects the modern MBT, the second - reflects the previous MBT; and the factorial matrix of students of the school of psychics reveals the most archaic of the three MBTs of mass consciousness; then the data structure of the models can be represented as follows.

1. Modern multicomponent MDT consists of blocks:
   - conservative therapy;
   - radical therapy;
   - traditional therapy, introjecting "external" and "internal" methods of treatment of the previous model;
   - therapy by psychic means (psychotherapy).
2. The previous two-component MDT consists of blocks of:
   - "external" methods of traditional therapy;
   - "internal" methods of traditional therapy.
3. The earliest of the compared, three-component-magical MBT consists of blocks:
   - spell-ritual magic therapy;
   - "external" methods of traditional therapy;
   - "internal" methods of traditional therapy.

It is fundamentally significant that the second and third archaic MDT were obtained with individual and socially conditioned regressive dynamics of the modern MDT. Consequently, modern MDT in a latent, mediated form contains previous MDT, which is possible only if MDT is a hierarchical, multi-level formation with the property of individual and social progressive historical development and regressive dynamics. So, MDT (both individual and social) is a systemic, hierarchical, multi-level formation, which can be represented as a hierarchical, multi-layer "spherical" structure, each layer-level of which corresponds to a certain historical stage in its development. The functioning of such a structure is determined by the activity of the highest, modern layer-level of the MDT. If the upper layer-level of the model of the effectiveness of medical care does not correspond to the individual, it is inactivated, with the transition of systemic functions to the MDT of the lower level. The correspondence of the subordinate levels of the MDT to certain historical epochs is probably not literal, only the most essential, key elements are preserved.

The assimilation by the individual of the MDT of mass consciousness, is provided by two mechanisms: "vertical" and "horizontal." The "vertical" mechanism plays a decisive role in the formation of the structure of the model, starting from the deep levels - at the first stages of socialization of the individual and is functioning in the general context of mastering culture, starting with its most archaized elements: myths, legends, fairy tales, signs, prejudices; in direct and indirect forms. The "horizontal" mechanism determines the detailed development of each individual level of the MDT and is based on the active interaction of the individual with the surrounding reality.

Three variants for the individual dynamics of MDT are possible.

The first variant is progressive dynamics of MDT, in which, due to the assimilation by individual from mass consciousness of modern scientific paradigms of pathogenesis and therapy, with formation of higher level of model, which takes on system-forming functions, integrating and transforming the functions of the underlying layers-levels.

The second variant is regressive dynamics, with inactivation, due to the ineffectiveness of the treatment of the highest level of MDT and the actualization of the underlying phylogenetically and ontogenetically preceding level of the model, which takes on system-forming functions.

The third variant - reactivation dynamics, in which due to positive outcome of therapy there occurs a restoration, of the functioning of the initially "external" level of MBT, deactivated by the previous regressive dynamics.

**2.5.2.5. Structure, Historical Development and Dynamics of Mass Consciousness Model of Disease and Therapy.**

Analyzing the structure and dynamics of the MDT, it is necessary to recognize the systemic unity, identity of the such models of individual and general mass consciousness. The MDT presents a systemic block in the structure of mass consciousness, its general model of the world, therefore, it must preserve the basic principles of its organization. So, we can assume that mass consciousness represents a hierarchical, historically forming multilevel system, the functioning of which is determined by the activity of the system-forming "external" level. Mass consciousness, as a system, probably has the progressive, regressive, reactivation dynamics discussed above.

Social tension, crisis from the position of the hierarchical system of mass consciousness can be considered as a discrepancy between the conditions of social life and the standards of the "external" level of the system, which should, according to our model, lead to a regressive dynamics of such a system, with the actualization of the historically previous level of mass consciousness, which takes system-forming functions. The disintegration processes that took place in the former USSR served as a vivid illustration of this provision. The regressive dynamics of the system of mass consciousness during social tension encompasses its highest level as a whole, deactivating all systemic blocks, including MDT. Mass interest in various forms of archaic, magical healing, extrasensory therapy, growing during the intensification of social disintegration, is natural. The first wave of telepsychotherapy by A. Kashpirovsky in 1989 [45, 46] in the 1990s was swallowed up by a flurry of "non-traditional," "folk healing" [12, 13, 47, 48, 50, 51, 52]. The development of such "non-traditional folk healing" during the period of social disintegration of 1988-1991. obeyed a certain pattern and proceeded in the direction of successive actualization: the verbal-symbolic (example of telepsychotherapy by AM Kashpirovsky [45, 46]); manual (A. Chumak [47, 48], D. Davitashvili [49] and many others); extrasensory-trance therapy, with the experience of moving in space (flights to “space,” to “planets of the hierarchy,” etc., in a trance state) [2]. In 1992-1993, the return of verbal-symbolic, spell-ritual healing (the coming of Maria Stephanie and sorcerers of Russia, the resumption of A. Kashpirovsky activities) took place. The noted dynamics of “folk healing” corresponds to the initial regressive dynamics of the magic block of the MDT during the collapse of the USSR, in the reverse order to the historical development of magical action (proceeding from the magic of movement in space to manual-object magic and verbal-symbolic magic), followed by the initial reactivation dynamics of the “model” with a return to verbal-symbolic magic during the initial stabilization of statehood in Russia [2, 39].

Based on the analysis of the experimental psychological material, as well as the socially conditioned dynamics of the MDT during the collapse of the USSR, we propose the following structure. Spherical, hierarchical MDT is represented by three main layers-levels.

1. The original, the most ancient, “nuclear” layer-level of the MDT is formed by magic therapy, which in turn includes three sublevels: the «deepest,” the most ancient sublevel of therapy by magical movement in space; next - manual (manual-manipulative-subject) magic therapy; historically the later, “external” sublevel of verbal-symbolic magical therapy.
2. The second, “intermediate” layer-level of the MDT is formed by traditional therapy, which distinguishes the opposing “external” and “internal” methods of therapy.
3. The third, modern, “superficial” layer-level of MDT includes conservative therapy, radical therapy, therapy with psychic means.

Moreover, the blocks of conservative and radical therapy of the outer layer-level are genetically related to the layer-level of traditional “external” and “internal” therapy, while the block of therapy with psychic means - with the layer-level of magic therapy, which is revealed during the regressive dynamics of MDT.

It should be noted that the actualization of archaic MBT took place earlier in the historical past, preceding and accompanying major social upheavals. So, on the eve of the Great French Revolution, the famous Anton Mesmer treated patients with "animal magnetism," and on the eve of October, the gloomy figure of the "healer" of the court and aristocratic Petersburg Grigori Rasputin "materialized."

The MBT of mass consciousness, relevant in the process of therapy, plays the role of a specific communicative "language" of the patient and the therapist. The correspondence of the representations of the patient and the therapist about the disease and its treatment leads to the establishment of psychotherapeutic contact, with the inclusion of individual psychological and biological mechanisms of psychotherapy. The degree to which the MDT context matches the psychological and biological changes of the patient is fundamentally insignificant.

### *2.5.3. The Mythological Nature of Mass Consciousness and Its Model of Disease and Therapy; Psychotherapeutic Aspect*

A comprehensive, experimental-psychological and historical analysis of the MBT of mass consciousness made it possible to: describe its historically formed multi-level structure and socially and personally determined dynamics; when studying the experimental and social regressive dynamics of MBT, to reveal the genetic affinity of surface and deep structures (for example, blocks of conservative and radical therapy of the outer layer-level with the layer-level of traditional "external" and "internal" therapy, and the block of therapy with psychic means - with a layer level of magic therapy). However, the momentary experimental regression of the formally rational "model" transforming into "externally - internal" and magical methods of therapy confirms the mythological essence of the modern model.

So, the MDT is a mythological entity, and its hierarchical structure and dynamics are the structure and dynamics of mythology [2, 38]. MDT is a mythological formation, and its hierarchical structure and dynamics are the structure and dynamics of mythology. Since the MDT as a system unit is included in the Model of World of mass consciousness, it is also a mythological formation. The lives of man and mankind are saturated with mythology.

The system of psychotherapy widespread in a certain society interacts satisfactorily with the actual MBT of mass consciousness. Such interaction is provided by adaptation to psychotherapy to the current "model," generation of a connecting script and its subsequent exploitation. Psychotherapy, which qualitatively corresponds to the current MDT, inevitably functions as a mythological system. Thus, in a social context, psychotherapeutic systems are essentially mythological systems. The socially conditioned dynamics of MDT generates the development of psychotherapy methods.

## 3. Psychological Component of Psychotherapy

Clinical psychotherapy is based on therapeutic communication between individuals or a group of individuals. Effective therapeutic communication triggers and maintains in the patient intrapsychic, intrapersonal mechanisms of psychotherapy, which provide the patient with the final result [2].

Psychological communication of psychotherapy is characterized by (a) a historically determined communicative style, (b) methodological goal-setting and instruments of therapy, (c) partial spontaneity of interpersonal interaction [2, 39].

The intrapsychic mechanisms of psychotherapy are obvious, since without them the therapeutic result is impossible. However, the obviousness of the latter is combined with the mirror-like pseudo-transparency of the "black box" of the psyche, in which the interested observer sees the desired content, which often presents a reflection of the applied communicative-interpersonal component of psychotherapy. The real intrapsychic mechanisms of the psychotherapeutic process are hidden "behind the mirror" of the individual's psyche and may, probably, not coincide with the methodically prescribed ones.

## 3.1. Psychological Communication in Psychotherapy

Psychological communication of psychotherapy is characterized by (a) a historically determined communicative style, (b) methodological goal-setting and instruments of therapy, (c) partial spontaneity of interpersonal interaction [2, 38].

### *3.1.1. Communicative Style of Psychotherapy*

The concept of communicative styles was formulated by the author in relation to hypnotherapy, in a comparative analysis of Directive hypnosis, Ericksonian hypnosis and the author's method of Universal Hypnotherapy [53].

Communicative styles (of hypnotherapy) are determined by: (a) the approach to the use of the initial representations about the method of psychotherapy (hypnosis) among participants in therapeutic communication, (b) the peculiarities of the implementation of therapeutic communication at the verbal and non-verbal levels, (c) the ratio of the activities of the sides of psychotherapy (hypnotherapy) and (d) application of feedback by the therapist. It has been demonstrated that communicative styles of hypnotherapy are characterized by a natural historical sequence of appearance and development, from the Directive to EricksonianЖ hypnosis and, further, to Universal Hypnotherapy, since hypnotherapy translates historically relevant communicative styles of active interaction of the mass consciousness []. It has been demonstrated that communicative styles of hypnotherapy are characterized by a natural historical sequence of appearance and development, from the "Directive to Ericksonian hypnosis and, further, to Universal Hypnotherapy, since hypnotherapy translates historically relevant communicative styles of active influence of the mass consciousness []. Each communicative style has a characteristic profile of opportunities and limitations that work at the socio-psychological and psychological levels.

The concept of communicative style is applicable to any psychotherapy method. So, communicative styles are transferred to psychotherapy from everyday life, the historical dynamics of mass consciousness determines natural changes in therapeutic communication.

### *3.1.2. Methodological Goal-Setting and Instruments of Psychotherapy*

Psychotherapy as a methodology includes the methodological goal-setting and methodological instruments [2]. The methodological component is determined by: theories underlying the applied methodological approaches to psychotherapy; methodological approaches embodied in specific psychotherapeutic techniques and patterns. Each method of psychotherapy attaches paramount importance to this component; in practice, the general understanding of psychotherapy is reduced to it.

### *3.1.3. The Spontaneity of Interpersonal Interaction in Psychotherapy*

Despite the requirement to adhere to the therapeutic protocol, both sides of the therapeutic process are represented by living people, who inevitably bring an element of unique spontaneity to the methodically regulated process. Therefore, the spontaneous-communicative component characterizes the influence of the individual-personal characteristics of the participants in the psychotherapeutic process (therapist and patient) in their real communicative interaction on the results of psychotherapy. The influence of the characterological characteristics of the psychotherapist and his style of behavior on the results of psychotherapy has been widely studied earlier, is well known [2], and therefore is not the subject of our consideration.

## 3.2. The Intrapsychic Mechanisms of Psychotherapy

In the process of clinical psychotherapy, the patient learns and assimilates a lot of new information about himself, his disease, the applied therapy, he manages to therapeutically modify and stabilize the modified state, behavior that provide the final therapeutic result. Psychotherapy undoubtedly uses a variety of learning mechanisms that are an important part of the intrapsychic component of psychotherapy [61-68].

However, in the interests of presentation, the author will limit himself to mentioning the well-known mechanisms of learning, highlighting other, previously emitted and described by him intrapsychic mechanisms related to the system of psychological adaptation of the personality [2, 38, 54].

### *3.2.1. Study of the Intrapsychic Personal System of Psychological Adaptation*

In the 1980"s and 1990"s, we investigated the dynamics of the MMPI basic scales before and after identical group hypnotherapy for two samples of patients with various types of anxiety disorders [2, 38, 54] (Mixed Anxiety-Depressive disorder, ASD (Acute Stress Disorder), PTSD (Post Traumatic Stress Disorder) along with Dissociative and Somatoform disorders, OCD (Obsessive-Compulsive Disorder (N = 145). Another group represented Anxiety Disorders due to Cerebrovascular disorder (N = 51). The design of the research included: 1) clinical estimation of psychotherapy efficiency; 2) analyses of MMPI data (basic scales (validity (L, F, K) and clinical scales (I – Hypochondrosis, 2 – Depression, 3 – Hysteria, 4 – Psychopathic Deviate, 5 - Masculinity/Femininity, 6 - Paranoia, 7 – Psychasthenia, 8 – Schizophrenia, 9 – Hypomania and O – Social Introversion), at the beginning and at the end of psychotherapy; 3) statistical analysis (descriptive statistics; means; nonparametric statistics [Wilcoxon matched pairs test] along with factor analysis - principal components method with varimax rotation). For each clinical group of psychotherapy efficiency, we analyzed within the Factor analysis the initial data, final data and data on dynamics of psychotherapy (received by subtraction of final data from initial data).

Our study revealed two levels of the efficiency of psychotherapy: significant improvement of the condition (equivalent of full recovery) with a full and persistent reduction of clinical disorders), and improvement of conditions with only partial or unstable reduction of clinical disorders [2, 38, 54]. This research has shown that patients, who displayed either significant improvement or improvement of conditions, differ from the very beginning and that there are two types of dynamics that represent mechanisms of the therapeutic effect and final outcomes of psychotherapy.

### *3.2.2. The Model of Personal System of Psychic Adaptation*

We attributed positive dynamics of affective symptoms to the restoration of the Personal System of Psychic Adaptation (PSPA), which is the primary mechanism of positive change in cases of efficient psychotherapy for anxiety disorders. With regard to cognitive-behavioral parameters, the therapeutic dynamics were associated with developmental mechanisms of mostly supplementing and rebuilding the Personal System of Psychic Adaptation which is the primary therapeutic mechanism in cases of efficient psychotherapy for Anxiety Disorders Due to Cerebrovascular Disorder.

In the 1980"s, based on our research on outcomes from psychotherapy of anxiety and organic disorders, we described a Personal System of Psychological Adaptation (PSPA) [2, 38, 54, 55]. PSPA is a spontaneously activated homeostatic dynamic structure which forms during ontogenesis and creates a hierarchy of adaptive mechanisms ranging from the earliest, most primitive and typical (similar to Freudian ego-defenses like Regression, Replacement, etc., which are normal for early childhood) to mature, complex, individualized and personal ones which can be used as coping mechanisms. Hierarchical PSPA can be visualized as a spherical multilayered model (see Figure 1) involving the following components.

1. Concentric structure of levels of the hierarchical organization of adaptation mechanisms that form an expanding sphere around a "center" or the "Ego," "Self." The highest mature level of hierarchy of multi-layer level mechanisms of psychological adaptation has a capability of transforming the interactions between the underlying levels.

PSPA dynamics may express themselves in regressive, reactivating or of progressive (forming) transformations:

- In cases of regressive dynamics (where there is relative inactivation of the highest, mature level of mechanisms of psychological adaptation) the underlying levels, ontogenetically antecedent to it, become primarily active and assume the role of regulatory functions overriding more advanced functions; this results in reorganization of the system of radial and spherical connections, and development of a new emotional and behavioral patterns not present at the previous stages of PSPA ontogenesis. Regressive dynamics is potentially convertible.

2. Reactivation dynamics became possible after previous PSPA regressive dynamics; it involves restoration of function of initially top level of psychological adaptations and of PSPA "normal functioning," which has been disturbed by its previous regressive dynamics.
3. The formation of PSPA dynamics is possible through development of a higher level which would overcome insufficiency and defectiveness of previous psychological adaptations of underlying levels.

In cases of anxious maladaptation (but not much disintegration), weakening in higher levels of PSPA adaptative mechanisms causes lower levels of adaptive mechanisms to acquire greater behavioral significance. (An example may be the development of dissociative symptoms in persons without a history of dissociative disorders in combat situations).

According to our model, psychotherapeutic interventions [2, 38, 54, 55] are especially suitable for cases of anxiety disorders in which there is a potential weakening of the PSPA due to regressive activation of early ontogenic adaptation mechanisms (i.e., dissociative disorders, obsessive) but also to a PSPA deficit which is due to personality disorders or to organically based brain disorders.

Evidently, mechanisms of effective psychotherapy in cases of reversible psychogenic blocking and PSPA organically based deficit must be different. In instances of regressive dynamics of PSPA, "higher," "normal" levels of psychological adaptation are deactivated psychogenically (or underutilized), in the course of maladaptive functioning and the goal of psychotherapy is to facilitate their proper functioning again. In the case of deficit, the higher layer-level of PSPA which controls other functions needs to be developed for the first time and as a result of efficient psychotherapy, an opportunity for a normal psychic adaptation be formed. Thus, in psychotherapy for anxious disorders, we attempt to activate the adaptive capability of the personality with reference to its already existing (but not fully utilized) resourcefulness. By contrast, in psychotherapy of personality and organic disorders, the therapeutic efforts are similar to spontaneous developmental processes leading to formation of the PSPA hierarchy, which means that the patients need to acquire resources allowing for better adaptation. The submitted results of MMPI data complex statistical analysis well reflect the above-stated conceptualization.

The results of our empirical research on hypnotherapy outcomes have revealed that dynamics of efficient hypnotherapy with complete improvement in anxiety disorders is consistent with the mechanism of reactivation, and for organic disorders - with an idea of PSPA formation; whereas in cases of partial improvement, the psychological dynamics for anxious disorders corresponds to partial PSPA reactivation, and for organic disorders – to incomplete PSPA formation. In our previous publications [2, 38, 54], we hypothesized that such incomplete PSPA reactivation and formation comprise isolated elements of opposite mechanisms.

Consistent with the general resourcefulness model, our empirically based conclusion is that psychogenic blocking causes underutilization of resources. It also describes two different ways of personal reintegration which lead to recovery in cases of anxiety disorder. The first way of recovery, determined as PSPA reactivation, is more effective, simple and needs fewer resources. PSPA reactivation is believed to correspond to Celinski and Pilowsky [56] "activation of latent personal qualities." The second way, namely PSPA formation, may be less effective and needs expanding, an acquisition of resources as PSPA formation requires acquisition through learning of new adaptive skills. In both instances

(PSPA reactivation and PSPA formation), in the end the dynamic processes enable individuals to utilize their resourcefulness.

Research reveals the multidimensional nature (both culturally and personally based) of a psychological ability to maintain health and to prevent pathological disorders [57, 58, 56, 59, 60].

Important questions remain about how recovery is possible in cases of various illnesses, what is the difference between complete and partial spontaneous recovery and what is the role of therapy for anxiety and organic disorders? What role can resourcefulness and resilience play in initiating and promoting psychological and physiological changes in cases of different psychotherapy outcomes?

We can believe that initial differences, in cases of complete and partial recovery, are determined by the primary differences in resourcefulness (and probably, resilience). We hypothesized that utilization of resourcefulness (reactivation and formation) reflect qualitative differences between disorders, and probable differences in an individual's initial resilience, in that more resilient people react in psychotherapy by PSPA reactivation, but less initially resilient – would require PSPA formation. This hypothesis needs further research.

It is our current understanding that mechanisms of reactivation and formation of the PSPA, revealed in our research, support the theoretical constructs of Resourcefulness and Resilience underlying the processes of psychotherapeutic recovery in cases of anxiety and organic disorders. Mechanisms of PSPA Reactivation and Formation, lead to acquiring psychic stability after injury by mostly returning to the original state or by forming stable conditions again. In psychotherapeutic reality, both processes are always developing together, but one of them is dominant and the other is supplementary. Both mechanisms belong to the Resourcefulness domain. The mechanism of PSPA Reactivation is close to the Resourcefulness" activation of latent personal qualities, while the PSPA Formation mechanism is linked to Resourcefulness as an ability to acquire new skills.

The question is why, in some cases, the PSPA reactivation process is easy to initiate and in other cases, PSPA formation remains less predictable. On the one hand, in cases of initial psychological and physiological stability, which is blocked psychogenically, psychotherapy may stimulate the PSPA reactivation process; however, when initial psychological and physiological stability is lacking (such as in cases of organic disorders), there is a need for of PSPA formation through psychotherapy. Chronic disorders will also increase the probability that the focus of therapy should be on PSPA formation processes. Thus, our study suggests, that PSPA reactivation and PSPA formation, while belonging to the Resourcefulness domain, represent two primary dynamic patterns of recovery. Thus, the nature of the physiological basis of Resourcefulness requires further research.

# 4. Biological Component of Psychotherapy

The patient's participation in psychotherapy changes his consciousness, thinking, behavior on the basis of effective learning [61-68].

Analyzing the experimental data of the phenomenon of neurogenesis, we formulated the conclusion that successful psychotherapy should stimulate the process of neurogenesis in patients [69], now this assumption is supported [70]. In our study, it was shown that, mono-psychotherapy is able to help patients to overcome the states of anxiety and depression in anxiety disorders [71], which needs positive neurobiological changes.

The author is engaged in research on hypnosis and hypnotherapy [53], therefore his analysis of the biological mechanisms of psychotherapy is limited by this method and is applicable in relation to its essential analogues.

## 4.1. Biological Component of Hypnotherapy

In the 1980s and 1990s, the author conducted research on the biological effect of a course of hypnotherapy on the blood system, in relation to its clinical efficacy in anxiety disorders. The obtained clinical and experimental data revealed that hypnotherapy has a distinct, systemic, biological effect on the patient's organism [53]. The following was found.

1. Hypnotherapy activates the systemic (stress-) readaptation processes that are reflected in changes in neurohormonal and neurotransmitter secretions; activities of the immunological system; activation of protein, bilirubin, and cholesterol exchange; etc.
2. Hypnotherapy activates protein metabolism and activity of several enzyme systems of the organism. Hypnotherapy has a positive influence on the metabolism of bilirubin. The activation of cholesterol metabolism, characterized by a significant reduction of its concentration in the blood, has a significant clinical importance. The observed decrease of cholesterol concentration in blood, normalizing its metabolism in the process of hypnotherapy, means the restoration of activity of cell membranes, cells, organs, and tissues, slowing down their aging.

The stressful nature of hypnosis limits its therapeutic application, in that excessive intensity of hypnogenic stress may result in the maladaptation. Prolonged hypnotherapy may actually decrease and exhaust adaptable resources of an organism.

Of course, the data of hypnotherapy should not be mechanically transferred to all methods of psychotherapy. But there is no reason to exclude the presence of a spectrum of biological mechanisms of psychotherapy associated with learning, neurogenesis, readaptation.

# 5. Discussion. Three-Component, Structural-Dynamic Theory of Psychotherapy

Earlier we consistently analyzed the socio-psychological, individual-psychological, biological components of psychotherapy [2, 38].

The performed analysis allows to proceed to a systematic presentation of the three-component theory of psychotherapy, highlighting its main points.

1. The presence of social, psychological, biological components of human nature predetermine the presence of socio-psychological, psychological, biological components of psychotherapy, which determine the patterns and mechanisms of the psychotherapeutic process.

The primary basis of the socio-psychological component of psychotherapy is the MDT, which represents the system block of “Model of the World” of mass consciousness. The MDT of mass consciousness and an individual, being a historically developing hierarchical system, retains in a latent form previous information and is subject to socially conditioned and individual dynamics in progressive, regressive, reactivation variants.

The psychological component of the psychotherapeutic process is formed by communicative-interpersonal and intrapsychic components. We highlight ehe intrapsychic component of psychotherapy, that is described in the context of the system of psychological adaptation of the personality - a spontaneous homeostatic ontogenetically formed hierarchical structure, which includes adaptive mechanisms that are consistently formed from early primitive, typological, to complex individualized, personal, which have regressive, reactivation, progressive dynamics.

The biological component of psychotherapy includes a complex of neurophysiological, organismic mechanisms that ensure the processes of readaptation, successful learning (including neurogenetic ones).

2. The psychotherapeutic process is based on complex psychological interaction and is carried out at two related levels of: socio-psychological, cultural interaction; interpersonal interaction founded on actual communicative style, methodological goal-setting and instruments of therapy, partial spontaneous interpersonal interaction.

Psychotherapeutic interaction at the socio-psychological level uses a connecting script that coordinates the theoretical and methodological tools of psychotherapy with the actual MDT of the patient, client. The actual MDT of mass consciousness plays the role of the "language" of communication between the patient and the therapist. The psychotherapeutic method may correspond to the actual MDT completely, partially, or significantly differ from it. In the first case, the content of psychotherapy is understood and accepted by the patient initially and completely. In the second and third cases, when the content of psychotherapy does not correspond to the actual MDT, it becomes necessary to reconcile them. In such cases, the methods of psychotherapy, mainly at the beginning of work with the patient, use the presentation of a connecting script that fills the existing semantic, logical gaps between the applied therapy and MDT. The initial or achieved correspondence between the patient's MDT and the method of psychotherapy leads to the establishment of psychotherapeutic contact and includes individual psychological and biological mechanisms of psychotherapy, initiating the psychotherapeutic process.

3. The complex psychological interaction carried out in the course of the psychotherapeutic process generates and supports the systemic psychological and biological reactions of the individual to the psychotherapeutic action, including intrapsychic sanogenic mechanisms and a complex of organismic mechanisms (biological, neurophysiological, neurohormonal, etc.).

In addition to the obvious mechanisms of effective learning, our study of psychotherapy at the intrapsychic level reveals the mechanisms of reactivation and formation of SPA of the individual, or their combination.

We believe that at the biological level psychotherapy engages mechanisms of stress-readaptive optimization of disturbed biological (and neurobiological) indicators.

# Conclusion

The three-component theory of psychotherapy, developed over 20 years ago, focuses on significant, natural and, at the same time, spontaneous phenomena of human life at social, psychological, biological levels.

The most significant data are obtained on the phenomenon of mass consciousness, its mythological nature, regressive dynamics in dead-end situations. The author is inspired by the fact that the modern mass consciousness in a latent, indirect and generalized form preserves the entire historical totality of cultural representations about the world and man (from the Stone Age to the present day). And the deepening regressive dynamics of mass consciousness is capable of consistently updating the previous levels of perception of the world, up to the most ancient ones. For the first time, the possibility of regressive dynamics of an individual's ideas about illness and therapy in an experimentally created dead-end situation is shown.

Psychotherapy presents a secondary phenomenon in relation to the current mass consciousness, everyday culture, therefore, the connecting script of psychotherapy becomes its most important means, the effectiveness of which increases with conscious application.

Modern psychotherapy is based on psychological communication, in which the therapist, as the architect of the project, together with the patient build a therapeutic result. The mechanisms of reactivation and the formation of a system of psychological adaptation of the personality, which are triggered by the patient's psyche independently, based on the characteristics of the disorder and the resources of the psyche, which are empirically identified by the author and consistent with a positive psychotherapeutic approach, are fundamental and enrich the understanding of psychotherapy.

The biological mechanisms of psychotherapy are inevitable for its active forms, are universal and based on the mechanisms of fixing positive experience (learning) and readaptation.

At the beginning of the millennium, the author, at an international symposium on suggestion and suggestiveness (Krakow, 2002), introduced to Western colleagues the results of studies of mass consciousness during the period of social deadlock and its roles in social life and psychotherapy [72]. The obtained data did not arouse much interest, since they were perceived as a specifically Russian phenomenon. I wonder how they are perceived now, in 2020?

## REFERENCES


[1] Karvasarsky B. D. (1985) *Psychotherapy*. Moscow: Meditsina Publishing, 298 p. (in Russian).

[2] Tukaev R. D. (2007) *Psychotherapy: theories, structures, mechanisms* (2nd edition, revised and enlarged). Moscow, Medical Information Agency Publishing House, 392 p. (in Russian).

[3] Van Gennep, Arnold (1909). *Les rites de passage* [The Rites of Passage] (in French). Paris: Émile Nourry.

[4] Turner, Victor. 1967. Betwixt and Between: The Liminal Period in Rites de Passage. *The Forest of Symbols: Aspects of Ndembu Ritual.* Ithaca, NY: Cornell University Press.

[5] Alekseev N. A. (1984) *Shamanism of the Turkish-speaking peoples of Siberia* (experience of areal comparative study). Novosibirsk: USSR Academy of Sciences, Siberian Branch, Yakutsk Branch, Institute of Language, Literature and History. 232 p (in Russian).

[6] Basilov V. N. (1984) *Chosen of Spirits*. Moscow: Politizdat publishing house., 208 p (in Russian).

[7] Kenin-Lopsan M. B. (1987) *Ritual practice and folklore of Tuvan shamanism. Late 19th - early 20th century*. Novosibirsk: Nauka publishing house, 164 p (in Russian).

[8] Sagalaev A. M. (1991) *Ural-Altai mythology: Symbol and archetype*. – Novosibirsk: Nauka publishing house, 151 p (in Russian).

[9] Smolyak A. V. (1991) *Shaman: personality, functions, worldview:* (Peoples of the Lower Amur). Moscow: Nauka publishing house, 280 p. (in Russian).

[10] Zabylin M. (1880) *Russian people, its customs, rituals, traditions, superstitions and poetry*. Moscow: Ed. bookseller M. Berezin, 608 p (in Russian).

[11] Toren M. D. (1996) *Russian folk medicine and psychotherapy*. SPb., Litera Publishing house. - 496 p (in Russian).

[12] Stepanova N. I. (2000) *500 spells of Siberian healing*. Moscow, Ripol-Classic publishing house, 480 p (in Russian).

[13] Urengoy V. (1992) *Treatment of spoilage*. Voronezh, Voronezh Publishing house, 63 p (in Russian).

[14] Goltsman E. (1990) *The Evil Eye. A book about the customs and superstitions of the peoples of the world*. Moscow: Prometheus publishing house. - 64 p (in Russian).

[15] *Mythological Dictionary*. (1991) *Moscow: Soviet encyclopedia*, 736 p (in Russian).

[16] Frazer J. G. (2016) *The Golden Bough: A Study in Magic and Religion: A New Abridgement from the Second and Third Editions*. (Oxford World's Classics) Reissue Edition.

[17] Freud S. (1955) *Lines of Advance in Psycho-Analytic Therapy (1919): Standard Edition, Vol. 17*. London: Hogarth Press.

[18] Freud S. (1955) *Beyond the Pleasure Principle (1920): Standard Edition, Vol. 18*. London: Hogarth Press.

[19] Freud S. (1955) *Group Psychology and the Analysis of the Ego: Standard Edition. Vol. 18*. London: The Hogarth Press.

[20] Freud S. (1961) *The Ego and the Id (1923): Standard Edition, Vol. 19*. London, Hogarth Press.

[21] Freud S. (1963) *Introductory Lectures on Psycho-Analysis (1916): Standard Edition, Vol. 15*. London: Hogarth Press.

[22] Freud S. (1964) *New Introductory Lectures on Psycho-Analysis (1933): Standard Edition, Vol. 22*. London: Hogarth Press.

[23] Freud S. (1964) *Analysis Terminable and Interminable (1937): Standard Edition, Vol. 23*. London: Hogarth Press.

[24] Fairbairn W. R. D. (1952). *Psychoanalytic Studies of the Personality*. London: Routledge & Kegan Paul.

[25] Guntrip H. (1973) *Psychoanalytic Theory, Therapy, and the Self: A Basic Guide to the Human Personality in Freud*, Erikson, Klein, Sullivan, Fairbairn, Hartmann, Jacobson, and Winnicott. New York: Basic Books. 224 p.

[26] Winnicott, D. W. (1989). D. W. Winnicott: *Psycho-analytic explorations.* (C. Winnicott, R. Shepard & M. Davis, Eds.). Harvard University Press.

[27] Fairbairn W. R. B. (1954) *An object-relations theory of the personality.* New York: Basic Books.

[28] Beck, J. S. (1995). *Cognitive Therapy basics and beyond*. New York: The Guilford Press.

[29] Beck, A., Freeman, A., Davis, D., A., Pretzer, J., Fleming, B., Ottaviani, R., Beck, J. S., Simon, K., Padesky, C., Meyer, J., & Trexler, L., & Associates. (2004). *Cognitive therapy of personality disorders, 2nd ed.* New York: Guilford.

[30] Beck, J. S. (2011). *Cognitive behavior therapy: Basics and beyond.* 2nd ed. New York: Guilford.

[31] Myasishchev V. N. (1960) *Personality and neuroses.* Leningrad, Leningrad University Publishing House, 426 p (in Russian).

[32] Karvasarsky B. D. (1980) *Neuroses. A guide for doctors*. Moscow: Medicine Publishing House, 448 p (in Russian).

[33] Fromm E. (1962) *Beyond the chaims of illusion: Myenconter with Marx and Freud.* New York: Simon and Schuster.

[34] Fromm E. (1973) *The anatomy of human destructiveness*. New York, Holt, Rinehart and Winston.

[35] Fromm E. (1976) *To have or to be?* New York: Harper and Row.

[36] Fromm E. (1980) *Greatness and limitations of Freud's thought*. New York: Harper & Row.

[37] Marx K., Engels F. Works. T. 19. *Second edition*. M.: Publishing house of political literature, 1961, p. 376 - 377. (in Russian).

[38] Tukaev R. D. (1990) The medical component of mass consciousness. Dynamics in conditions of social tension. In: *Materials of All-Union conference "Sociology of socio-political problems of the renewal of socialism: regional aspects."* Ufa, p. 73-74 (in Russian).

[39] Tukaev R. D. (2003) *Psychotherapy: structures, mechanisms*. Moscow, Medical Information Agency, 296 p. (in Russian).

[40] Fransella, F. Bannister D. (2004) [1977]. *A manual for repertory grid technique (2nd ed.)*. Chichester, UK; Hoboken, NJ: John Wiley & Sons.

[41] Gaava Luvsan (1986) *Traditional and modern aspects of oriental reflexology*. - Moscow: Nauka Publishing House, 576 p (in Russian).

[42] Shchutsky Yu. K. (1993) *Chinese Classical Book of Changes: 2nd ed.* Moscow: Nauka Publishing House, 606 p (in Russian).

[43] Badmaev P. (1991) *Fundamentals of medical science in Tibet. Zhud-Shi*. M.: Nauka Publishing House, 256 p (in Russian).

[44] Ibn Sina Abu Ali (1994) *Canon of Medicine. Selected Sections. Part 1*. Moscow: Kommercheskiy vestnik Publishing House; Tashkent: Fan Publishing House, 400 p (in Russian).

[45] Kashpirovsky A. M. (1993) *Group non-specific psychotherapy*. Moscow: TEK Ltd, 232 p. (in Russian).

[46] Morgovsky A. (1990) *Sessions by A. Kashpirovsky*. Moscow: Prometheus publishing house, 47 p. (in Russian).

[47] Borodin V. (1989) *About Alan Chumak without speculation*. Medical newspaper, N 103 (in Russian).

[48] Grimak L. P. (1994) *The Magic of the Biofield. Energy-informational treatment*. Moscow: Republic publishing house, 448p (in Russian)

[49] Davitashvili D. (1988) *I listen to my hands*. Moscow: Physical culture and sport publishing house, 191 p (in Russian).

[50] Zaitseva V. (1991) *An appointment with a... physicist*. Medical newspaper, N 18 (in Russian).

[51] Konovalova I. (1990) *Medicine grew out of witchcraft*. Medical newspaper, N 93 (in Russian).

[52] Krasnopolskaya I., Veretennikova I. (1990) *Order of sorcerers*. Soviet youth, No. 59 (in Russian).

[53] Tukaev R. D. (2006) *Hypnosis; Phenomenon and Clinical Application*. Moscow: Medical Information Agency, 448 p (in Russian).

[54] Tukaev R. Research on the effectiveness of the universal hypnotherapy model. In: Selinski MJ, Gow KM, editors. *Continuity versus Creative Response to Challenge: The Primacy of Resilience and Resourcefulness in Life and Therapy*. New York: Nova Science Publishers; 2011. pp. 499-520 (In Russian).

[55] Tukaev R. D. (1988) The mechanisms of psychological defense in emotional stress psychotherapy. In the book: *The Eighth All-Union Congress of Neuropathologists, Psychiatrists and Narcologists: Abstracts*. Moscow, 1988; v. 3: pp. 506-507 (In Russian).

[56] Celinski, M. J., Pilowsky, J. (2008). Measuring Resilience to Psychological Outcomes of Natural Disasters. More questions than answers. In K. Gow, and D. Paton. (Eds.), *The Phoenix of Natural Disasters: Community Resilience*. New York: Nova Science Publishers, pp. 73-86.

[57] Antonovsky A. (1980) *Health, stress, and coping*. Jossey-Bass Publishers, 255 p.

[58] Wolff A. C., Ratner P. A. (1999) Stress, social support, and sense of coherence. *West. J. Nurs. Res.* vol. 21, N 2, pp. 182–197.

[59] Celinski, M. J., and Gow, K. M. (2005). Trauma Clients: How understanding disintegration can help to reveal resourcefulness of the self. *Australian Journal of Clinical and Experimental Hypnosis*, 33, 195-217.

[60] Celinski M. J., Allen LM. (2011) Resourcefulness as the art of succeeding. In: Selinski MJ, Gow KM, editors. *Continuity versus Creative Response to Challenge: The Primacy of Resilience and Resourcefulness in Life and Therapy*. New York: Nova Science Publishers; pp. 343–358.

[61] Grosjean B. (2005) From synapse to psychotherapy: the fascinating evolution of neuroscience. *Am J Psychother.*; v. 59 (3), pp. 181-197.
[62] Dannehl K., Rief W., Euteneuer F. (2019) Effects of cognitive behavioural therapy on verbal learning and memory in major depression: Results of a randomized controlled trial. *Clin Psychol Psychother.,* v. 26 (3), pp. 291-297.
[63] Scherf N., Spruit E., Köhler S., Kronenberg G. (2019) Avoiding the Traps of Thought: The Relevance of Language and Rules for Acceptance and Commitment Therapy. *Fortschr Neurol Psychiatr.*, v. 87 (8), pp. 412-420.
[64] Minear M., Coane J. H., Boland S. C., Cooney L. H., Albat M. (2018) The benefits of retrieval practice depend on item difficulty and intelligence. *J Exp Psychol Learn Mem Cogn.*, v. 44 (9), pp 1474-1486.
[65] Kuei T., Tsai M., McLeod H. J., White R. G., Kanter J. (2019) Using the primary process emotional-behavioural system to better meet patient needs in psychotherapy. *Clin Psychol Psychother.*, v. 26(1), pp. 55-73.
[66] Boutelle K. N., Bouton M. E. (2015) Implications of learning theory for developing programs to decrease overeating. *Appetite*, v. 93, pp. 62-74.
[67] Marić N. P., Jašović-Gašić M. (2010) Neurons on the couch. *Psychiatr Danub.*, v. 22 (4), pp 484-487.
[68] Weersing V. R., Weisz J. R. (2002) Mechanisms of action in youth psychotherapy. *J Child Psychol Psychiatry*, v. 43 (1), pp 3-29.
[69] Tukaev R. D. (2008) The phenomenon of adult brain neurogenesis in experimental and clinical studies; aspects of etiopathogenesis of mental disorders, psychopharmacotherapy and psychotherapy. *Social and Clinical Psychiatry..* v. 18 (2), pp 96-102 (In Russian).
[70] Gorman J. M. (2016) *Combining Psychodynamic Psychotherapy and Pharmacotherapy. Psychodyn. Psychiatry.*, v. 44 (2), pp. 183-209.
[71] Tukaev R. D., Kuznecov V. E. (2015) Cognitive-oriented psychotherapy for anxiety disorders in a controlled trial. *Social and Clinical Psychiatry. vol. 25* (2), pp. 55-64 (in Russian).

[72] Tukaev R. D. (2003) Mass consciousness "Illness and Therapy Model" structure and dynamics as a component of suggestibility and placebo phenomena. *The 4th International Symposium on Suggestion and Suggestibility. Book of abstracts*. Krakow, Poland.

## BIOGRAPHICAL SKETCH

***Rashit Tukaev***

**Affiliation**: Department of Psychotherapy and Sexology, Russian Medical Academy of Continuous Professional Education, Ministry of Healthcare of the Russian Federation, Moscow, Russia.

**Education**: Bashkir State Medical Institute, Faculty of Medicine (1977); candidate of medical sciences (1987), doctor of medical sciences (1999).

**Research and Professional Experience**: Senior Researcher and Leading Researcher at the Ufa Research Institute of Ecology and Occupational Medicine (1987-2001), Leading Researcher at Moscow Scientific Research Institute of Psychiatry Ministry of Health (2001-2019), professor of Department of Psychotherapy and Sexology, Russian Medical Academy of Continuous Professional Education, Ministry of Healthcare (2010-2020). Research activity: ecology (environmentally related diseases, mechanisms); methods of psychotherapy of anxiety disorders, theoretical analyze of psychotherapy, hypnosis, methods of hypnotherapy.

**Professional Appointments**: the member of the Russian Society of Psychiatrists, Professional Psychotherapeutic League (Russia), EAP, ESH, ISH, President of the Association of Experts in the Field of Clinical Hypnosis (Russia).

**Publications from the Last 3 Years**:

1. Tukaev R., Kuznetsov V. (2019) Criteria and Predictors of Effectiveness of Psychotherapy of Anxiety Disorders. *Psychiatry, psychotherapy and clinical psychology, v 10*, № 2, pp 201-302.
2. Tukaev R. D. (2018) Synthetic model of the personality for psychotherapy. *Social and clinical psychiatry*, vol. 28 № 2, pp 55-62.
3. Tukaev R., Sryvkova K., Antipova O., Kuznetsov V., Stefanov G. (2017) Dynamics of Heart Rate Variability in hypnosis in healthy young men and women. *Psychiatry psychotherapy and clinical psychology*, v. 8, № 4, pp 484-498.

In: Psychotherapy
Editor: Hayley Boyd
ISBN: 978-1-53618-877-6


*Chapter 2*

# From Caterpillar to Butterfly: Stages of the Novice Therapist

***Eleanor E. Beale*[*]*, MA, Stephanie H. Gomez, BS and James Overholser, PhD***
Department of Psychological Sciences,
Case Western Reserve University, Cleveland, OH, US

## Abstract

The early stages of a career as a psychotherapist can be exhilarating yet challenging. When first learning how to be a psychotherapist, graduate students must juggle a flood of information about psychotherapy while simultaneously forming their own identity as a therapist. The present chapter describes the general stages experienced by novice therapists. 1) Understanding the challenges and fears associated with therapy, 2) Learning the basics of being in the room with a client, 3) Integrating evidence-based practice with common skills, 4) Developing a therapeutic orientation and identity, 5) Continuing the professional evolution. Psychotherapy relies on a supportive bond that has been based in a fiduciary relationship and hope. Over the course of therapy, both

[*] Corresponding Author's E-mail: eleanor.beale@case.edu.

therapist and client can learn, change, and grow in important ways. For the novice psychotherapist, the amount of information and knowledge ahead can be simultaneously exciting and daunting. The presented notions are derived through combining the perspectives of a clinician with 30 years of experience in clinical practice with the perspectives of current graduate students at different levels of training. These guidelines are meant to identify and validate the common early stages of becoming a therapist.

**Keywords:** novice therapist, psychotherapy training, professional development

## Introduction

Growing into the role of a psychotherapist is often a circuitous path and a dynamic process. Numerous theories, guidelines, and research studies have examined the topic of developing as a psychotherapist. However, none of these resources can fully capture the experience. To a certain extent, each novice therapist must go through an individual journey, starting as one version of a psychology student and ending as a trained psychotherapist, with an infinite number of adjustments along the way.

Every therapist experiences a unique process along their journey of professional development, but there are several identifiable stages of progress that ebb and flow along the way. These stages can be compared to the life cycle of a caterpillar growing into a butterfly. In many ways, the full cycle from caterpillar to butterfly may be repeated across the career of a psychologist, capturing the personal and professional growth that evolves over time. The timeline may fluctuate, but each novice therapist must contend with the different stages of change that emulate the metamorphosis from sheltered caterpillar into soaring butterfly.

The first stage of life for a butterfly is an egg (Thomas 2014). These eggs come in different shapes and sizes, and contain a tiny, growing caterpillar. Similarly, every therapist begins their professional journey as a training student, with varying levels of relevant knowledge and experience. Each therapist begins with the shared goal of learning psychology, although they may focus on different types of therapy or client populations. There are many choices for a novice therapist to make, and these choices come with excitement, fear, and indecision.

The second stage of life for a butterfly is the caterpillar, or larva. The main activity during the larval stage is consumption, typically beginning with eating the very leaf onto which it was born. Caterpillars grow rapidly through a process called molting, during which the insect sheds its outgrown skin on several different occasions. Similarly, during graduate school, the goal of a developing therapist is to consume, i.e., absorbing new ideas through graduate coursework, supervised clinical services, and discussions with a mentor. With each new class, each new client, and each new supervisor, the novice therapist molts, grows, and evolves.

The third stage of life for a butterfly is the pupa, or chrysalis. Within the shell of the pupa, the caterpillar goes through a metamorphosis in which the original structure of tissue, limbs, and organs of the caterpillar is completely transformed. This may be the most obtuse part of developing as a psychologist. A great deal of metamorphosis occurs from the beginning of graduate school through the later stages of a career. Yet, there is change and restructuring in all arenas of becoming a therapist; some more obvious and some more subtle. During this time, the professional identity and personal life of the young therapist evolves into a unified whole.

The fourth and final life stage is the adult butterfly. Upon emergence from the chrysalis, a butterfly must rest to allow for proper blood flow to develop throughout its wings. Eventually, the novice therapist emerges as a licensed, skilled, and seasoned psychotherapist. The professional evolution does not stop there, as it is up to each psychotherapist to continue growing, restructuring, and improving to a newer form and mature identity.

The aim of this chapter is to highlight recognizable stages of growing from a novice therapist into a seasoned clinician. Bolstered by experience of the authors who fall at different stages of training, the chapter is meant to describe some of the less formal processes involved in professional development. Starting with the apprehension involved in clients for the first time, we discuss understanding the challenges and fears associated with therapy. Then, we address the experience of learning the basics of building a therapeutic alliance. Next, we focus on struggles involved when attempting to integrate evidence-based practice with common clinical skills, balancing education and research with hands-on experience. We reflect on developing a therapeutic orientation and establishing a professional identity as an exciting but conflicting process. Finally, we comment on the continuation of professional development across the career of a therapist.

## Understanding the Challenges and Fears Associated with Therapy

After completing the relevant coursework, reading countless journal articles, and role-playing with colleagues to prepare for one's first client, many students do not feel ready to step into the role of "therapist." There is nothing quite like being in the room with a client for the first time, and not knowing what to say (Cynkar and Schwartz 2007). Novice therapists are typically overwhelmed with both excitement and apprehension at the beginning of their careers, but the most common feelings amongst novice therapists are fear and anxiety stemming from self-doubt (Dong et al. 2018). Although these feelings are justified, as there are many unique challenges that new therapists face when beginning to see clients, most novice therapists are better prepared for this task than they feel. The more the novice understands what lies ahead, the more they can feel empowered to face their fears with courage and confidence. Acknowledging and understanding the various fears that are faced by novice therapists is the first step towards conquering the fears, and leads to professional growth.

One of the most basic challenges that novice therapists face is their limited knowledge about psychotherapy in general. Novice therapists have the unique challenge of practicing therapy even though they have not completed their training programs (Skovholt and Rønnestad 2003). They may still be familiarizing themselves with basic issues regarding diagnostic assessment and different types of psychopathology. Novice therapists may be learning various therapeutic techniques, and sharpening their clinical interviewing skills. There may be strategies or concepts they do not fully understand. Therefore, a novice therapist may be more likely to feel "stuck" during a session because they do not know how to steer the conversation to be more therapeutically productive. They may feel that their lack of knowledge inhibits their ability of being the best therapist they can be for their client. However, novice therapists should realize that research supports the effectiveness of trainees providing psychotherapy. A recent study conducted at a university department psychology training clinic in Sweden showed that graduate students can provide cognitive behavioral therapy that produces significant reductions in client symptoms (Hiltunen, Kocys, and Perrin-Wallqvist 2013). Results showed that clients who completed therapy with their novice therapist were able to reduce their symptoms and improve their quality of life. Furthermore, research has found that accumulated years of experience working as a therapist is not a significant predictor of client improvement (Goldberg et al. 2016). A longitudinal study found that therapists did not improve with additional experience, whether experience was based on the number of clients treated across the person's career or based on the number of years since the therapist obtained their terminal degree (Goldberg et al. 2016). Thus, novice therapists should trust their abilities and not compare their performance to fictionalized images of an idealized therapist.

For a novice therapist, common sources of stress include performance anxiety, evaluation from superiors, managing emotional boundaries, lack of confidence, inexperience with case conceptualization, glamorized expectations about psychotherapy, and an ongoing need for helpful mentorship (Skovholt and Rønnestad 2003). Although being a student with a limited knowledge base can be perceived as a challenge or limitation, there are also some benefits to treating clients while still participating in a graduate training program. Therapy students typically have access to many resources through their programs: supervisors, faculty, relevant journal articles, peer support of other novice therapists, professional colloquiums, and graduate classes that may be directly related to current clients. These resources can be extremely useful, especially for a young clinician who is able to apply this knowledge to their clinical work.

All therapists strive to become better clinicians, and may look to improve their therapeutic skills throughout their careers. However, for some, the desire to improve as a therapist may be rooted in feelings of insecurity and self-doubt. Among a sample of 155 psychotherapy practitioners, feelings of doubt about their own therapeutic effectiveness was one of the most commonly reported personal issues in therapists (Mahoney 1997). Novice therapists commonly possess a lack of confidence in their therapeutic skills. This is partially due to their lack of experience, and partially due to their tendency to second-guess their decisions during a therapy session, frequently asking themselves: "Did I say the right thing?"; "Did I properly execute that technique?"; and "Maybe I am not cut out to be a therapist?" Although it is beneficial to be aware of one's weaknesses and to strive to do better, there is a difference between self-awareness and self-doubt. While a therapist's self-awareness can be beneficial in terms of building rapport and sensitivity to the therapeutic process, a therapist's self-doubt may disrupt the flow of a session. Self-doubt and insecurity may create feelings of anxiety, depression, worry, or burnout in the therapist (Truell 2001), which can lead to decreased effectiveness during therapy sessions. Novice therapists should remember that psychotherapy relies on a strong personal relationship, with core elements including a gentle supportive style, genuine feelings of concern and compassion for the client, and a willingness to listen to anything the client wants to discuss. These are not abstract technical skills but good qualities that underlie any intimate and supportive relationship. When novice therapists are able to relax and relate to the client as two people having a thoughtful discussion, the session will flow easily. By trusting the basic elements of empathy, genuineness, and unconditional positive regard (Rogers 1957), psychotherapy becomes a simple supportive bond between a caring professional and an individual in a state of distress.

Feelings of self-doubt do not necessarily indicate inadequate performance. Even seasoned clinicians may report feelings of insecurity about their ability to help a client. In fact, feelings of doubt are helpful because they can push the therapist to learn, grow, and improve in the therapy they provide. In a qualitative study involving semi-structured interviews with practicing therapists, Theriault et al. (2009) found that feelings of incompetence had both positive and negative effects. Therapists reported that when they had feelings of incompetence, they would compensate by changing the pace of therapy, increasing self-disclosure, allowing more silence, and making other modifications to improve their techniques. However, they also reported that feelings of incompetence led to distraction during sessions, disengagement from the therapeutic process, and even detachment from the client (Thériault, Gazzola, and Richardson 2009). Novice therapists can use a moderate amount of self-doubt as a strength while acknowledging that too much can interrupt therapeutic flow. Thus, self-doubt is useful at any stage of one's career because it can push for critical self-evaluation, honest awareness of strengths and weaknesses, and ongoing efforts for improvement.

Novice therapists who experience self-doubt or insecurity during their sessions may feel isolated because these feelings are rarely discussed amongst mental health professionals. They may feel alone in their experiences, leading to compounded stress and emotional exhaustion. However, these feelings are quite common in the professional community and are part of the development into a professional. Acceptance can be a powerful tool to combat these fears in the novice therapist. It is a myth that seasoned psychotherapists never make mistakes. Even supervisors may say the "wrong" thing in a session (Topor et al. 2017). Novice therapists may be able to reduce their self-imposed pressure by accepting mistakes as a part of the learning process. Novice therapists can support each other regarding their feelings of self-doubt and opposed feelings of incompetence. Everyone makes mistakes. The important thing is to learn from that mistake so it becomes less likely to happen again.

Novice therapists want to help their clients and make changes so that the presenting problems begin to subside. The novice often aims for full remission from a psychiatric disorder, working towards the goal of "curing" their clients. This mindset is based on the Therapist

Responsibility Model (Ellis 2004), which is rooted in the medical model, and maintains that the therapist is the "knowledgeable expert" who takes on the role of "healer" to "cure" the client. This outlook is problematic for a number of reasons. First, novice therapists put an undue amount of pressure on themselves to reach high goals for their clients, and thereby place pressure on the clients. The novice therapist may expect to see measurable improvement in a timely manner, making the therapist impatient. However, it seems useful to remember that most psychiatric disorders involve lifelong struggles that disrupt the client's functioning every day (Keyes 2007). Clients do not wake up one day completely healed of their psychiatric disorders. However, they can make small amounts of progress each week. More importantly, clients can be helped to develop the coping skills needed to manage their symptoms on a daily basis. Seeing client improvement should be the goal, rather than seeing the client be cured. Therapy can be a slow process with small changes that accrue across multiple sessions. Therapists must learn to be patient, supporting small but progressive improvements that may occur across multiple sessions.

Second, when a novice therapist is focused on curing the client, they may rush through a treatment plan without allowing adequate time to build rapport. Many aspects of psychotherapy require time, patience, and persistence. Therapy often includes elements of exploration, acceptance, and understanding of clients' experience (Rihacek and Roubal 2018). Graduate training can help novice therapists learn the importance of the therapeutic alliance as the foundation for effective therapy. An overemphasis on wanting to do the right thing in therapy could reduce time spent on understanding the client. If the therapist adheres to a strict schedule in order to reach a predetermined goal, they may miss some key elements required for lasting improvement.

Finally, a focus on curing a client may result in low quality therapy. The therapist might experience anxiety, stress, and burnout when they are unable to meet their goal. Instead, novice therapists can view therapy as a collaborative process, in which therapist and client work together to promote change. It is helpful for novice therapists to be flexible in their goals, processes, and strategies, and to avoid setting deadlines on any client goals. Therapists can identify small improvements that can accumulate into in large victories over time. Therapy is not a race, and different people require different amounts of time to see improvement. Due to a range of demographic and clinical factors, clients might get worse before they get better, and they will most likely relapse multiple times before reaching full remission (Adebiyi et al. 2018). In fact, some clients might never reach full remission. Novice therapists can encourage clients in a supportive, non-judgmental manner on their path towards recovery. Therapists should not blame themselves if progress is slow or recovery is incomplete. Psychotherapy is not a predetermined process with a final cure, but an ongoing process of gradual change that varies with each client.

When they start seeing clients, novice therapists are often concerned about suicide risk. There are issues relating to liability and malpractice that must be taken into account when treating suicidal clients (Jobes and Berman 1993). Every institution that provides outpatient therapy should have a protocol in place for how to assess suicide risk and handle a suicide crisis. It is vital that novice therapists understand and follow these protocols when necessary. These protocols ensure that clients are not sent home if they pose imminent risk of harming themselves. Additionally, documentation of these protocols provides legal protection for the therapist and the institution (Simpson and Stacy 2004). Novice therapists can always call their supervisors if they are unsure of how to handle a particular situation. The therapist should take steps to ensure the safety of the client and document these strategies in their notes. Across their career, about 25 percent of therapists experience a client dying by suicide (Veilleux 2011). More likely, some clients will need to be hospitalized for suicidal ideation or intent. However, if a novice therapist experiences a client's suicide and they have followed appropriate protocols, their legal liability should be contained. First, the therapist should follow the necessary protocol to ensure the client's safety. Second, a client's suicide is not indicative of their effectiveness as a therapist or their worth as a clinician. Third, many other therapists have been in similar situations and there are resources for dealing with a such a tragedy.

Supervisors can help novice therapists as they manage these fears and expectations about beginning therapy with clients. Prevalence of physical and mental health symptoms are higher among clinical psychology graduate students than the general population (Rummell 2015). There is a great deal of work involved when learning to be a therapist. Novice therapists must balance classwork, research goals, and clinical training while juggling pressure from other personal and academic responsibilities. Supervisors can help trainees to decrease their tendencies for self-criticism and increase self-compassion in hopes of preventing the early stages of burnout (Richardson, Trusty, and George 2020). Supervisors can check with graduate students about life activities and relaxation skills outside school. Supervisors serve as a source of inspiration in addition to a resource for learning about how to conduct therapy (Maruniakova, Rihacek, and Roubal 2017). Particularly in the early stages of training, a clinical supervisor may be the main source of support for a novice therapist. Checking in with novice therapists about fears and boosting coping skills will improve trainee stability. Supervisors can reflect on their own struggles when first learning to be a therapist, and appreciate how current training has become aggravated by the influx of information and numerous advances in psychological theories. Supervisors can minimize any unrealistic expectations for their trainees. When supervisors can provide a safe and supportive environment for clinical case discussions, the novice therapist can feel free to express their worries, struggles, and potential errors. The supervisor aims to balance the goals of providing sound training for the novice while also ensuring high quality of care for the client (Overholser 2004). Trainees can learn to use their time in supervision in order to request guidance and support when needed. Trainees should trust their supervisor to be a skilled and tolerant mentor who can help guide the trainee whenever difficult situations arise in psychotherapy sessions or away from work. Furthermore, it can empower the trainee to seek support and gain assistance from a more senior psychologist, without feeling interrogated by a superior.

## LEARNING THE BASICS OF BEING THE THERAPIST WITH A REAL CLIENT

Novice therapists have a variety of fears when they first start seeing clients. Beyond these fears is the reality of what actually happens during therapy sessions. The best way to know what it is like to be a therapist is to work as a therapist. Learning the basics of therapy is comparable to the enormous amount of consumption that occurs when a caterpillar begins to grow. Part of this growth involves reading books and journal articles about some of the established therapeutic interventions. However, a larger portion of growth involves feeling comfortable with being the therapist in the room, responsible for the care and well-being of the client. There are key elements of the therapy process that are applicable to any therapeutic orientation.

Arguably the most important thing when conducting psychotherapy is the relationship between the therapist and the client. Many elements go into the development of a strong therapeutic alliance (Lavik et al. 2018). When first meeting a client it is more important to start building trust and rapport, and less important to have an expert amount of knowledge on a particular therapeutic orientation. Focusing on rapport and supportive listening may help to decrease the novice therapist's self-induced pressure to initiate change. Understanding the importance of the therapeutic relationship encourages the therapist to dedicate a substantial amount of time toward building rapport. The act of building rapport does not require any nuanced training or complex skills, rather it involves simply being an empathetic person who listens and instills hope in the client. Most people will not feel comfortable disclosing their deepest emotional struggles to a person whom they just met. Therefore, allowing the client to gradually develop trust in the therapist is key for self-disclosures and open discussions in treatment. Measurable improvement in client symptoms may not be seen for months after treatment has started, and so novice therapists can take solace in the fact that the first few sessions will be focused on building the therapeutic relationship.

Part of building rapport involves understanding the client's expectations for therapy. Clients have described experiencing judgment from the therapist and not being ready to discuss a particular topic as moments of hindrance during treatment (Swift, Tompkins, and Parkin 2017). Novice therapists may emphasize the collaborative nature of therapy, the value of individualized goals for treatment, and the likely ups and downs over the course of therapy. The novice therapist can realize that therapy will progress differently with each particular client.

A key aspect of building rapport with clients is being fully engaged throughout all moments of the therapy sessions. Novice therapists must enter their sessions with the mindset that this hour is dedicated to their work with the client. As novice therapists are usually students, they typically have a myriad of other deadlines and responsibilities on any given day, and it can be difficult to set aside thoughts of their other obligations. However, being fully present and engaged with the client provides a solid foundation for a respectful and trusting therapeutic relationship. Novice therapists can be self-aware of their own distractions, and direct their focus back onto the client (Nutt Williams 2008). Additionally, nonverbal behaviors and body language are extremely important for novice therapists to be aware of during their sessions, as these factors can influence the therapeutic relationship. Novice therapists can rely on using open and welcoming body language, such as maintaining good posture, relaxing the arms and legs, smiling, and speaking with a warm tone of voice. High levels of high eye contact and forward leaning posture have been found to enhance perceived therapist empathy and therapeutic alliance (Dowell and Berman 2013). Nonverbal behaviors can convey that the therapist is focused on the client, and will not be distracted by external stimuli. Finally, asking questions expresses interest and curiosity in what the client is saying, and shows that that the therapist is trying to understand and help the client. A strong therapeutic alliance has been found to include asking questions, making encouraging comments, identifying and reflecting back on the client's feelings, making positive comments about the client, and validating the client's experiences (Duff and Bedi 2010). Although these skills may seem basic and self-explanatory, they can easily be forgotten while trying to provide treatment. If novice therapists get into the habit of using these skills, it will become a natural part of their therapeutic technique over time.

When the therapist is fully engaged and focused on the discussion, it becomes easier to establish empathy and to validate the client's feelings. Empathy is a significant predictor of treatment outcomes in psychotherapy (Elliott et al. 2018). Especially in the first few therapy sessions, clients may disclose a mix of information regarding relationship issues, past traumatic events, and other current life stressors. By acknowledging that clients have a right to feel the way they do, the therapist supports the client and the client's subjective reactions. Validation and empathy are some of the most basic ways that novice therapists can show support for their clients. In contrast, it can be quite damaging to the therapeutic alliance if the therapist invalidates the client's feelings, even when unintentional. It is important to appreciate the importance of validation and empathy for developing a strong therapeutic alliance.

In addition to building rapport, the novice therapist begins therapy with the underlying goal of instilling hope for positive change arising from therapy. The presence of hope can have a profound impact on therapeutic outcomes, including treatment adherence, treatment satisfaction, and general therapeutic effectiveness (Irving et al. 2004, Larsen, Edey, and Lemay 2007). Increasing client hope means encouraging the client to believe that things can get better and therapy can help them make positive changes. However, instilling hope does not necessarily involve explicitly discussing hope with the client or claiming that things will definitely improve, as this could actually become a hindrance to treatment (Larsen, Edey, and Lemay 2007). Rather, novice therapists can instill hope by increasing the client's belief that therapy is effective and the therapist is competent. Unfortunately, novice therapists may doubt whether they can actually help their clients. Hope within the therapist comes with experience, and at the novice stage may relate to an understanding of the research evidence that documents the effectiveness of an intervention. The more hope that a therapist has in their own abilities to help their clients, the greater likelihood that the client will actually improve (Coppock et al.

2010). Many clients immediately feel a sense of hope in therapy simply because there is a supportive and empathetic person that wants to help them. The fact that a client has sought therapy is evidence of the client's baseline level of hope. Overall, instilling hope in clients can derive from a therapist who provides a sense of validation, expresses empathy, and feels secure in their own abilities to help the client.

Novice therapists benefit from embracing each session with a client as a learning experience. There are an abundance of opportunities for trainees to learn about the individual client as well as about themselves by noticing reactions, bonding moments, and chances for new perspectives. When facing ongoing evaluation regarding their skills as a therapist, it is easy to assume that all feedback is factual. Part of developing as a novice therapist involves learning to incorporate valuable feedback received from supervisors while also developing your own style of therapy.

Supervisors and faculty members who are teaching clinical courses can help to instill confidence and hope in novice therapists. Trainees can be reminded that even expert therapists had to start as a novice with their first client. Supervisors can explain basic therapy skills including instruction, modeling, practice, feedback, and reflection on experiences (Hill, Stahl, and Roffman 2007). Keeping a non-judgmental dialogue with novice therapists about what goes well and what can be improved in therapy may reduce initial concerns about being observed and evaluated by a supervisor. Supervisors can remind themselves that early stages in training involve constant appraisal from superiors (Dong et al. 2018). Praise is just as important as criticism throughout clinical supervision. Furthermore, supervisors can set their expectations to align with the developmental level of the trainee (Rønnestad et al. 2018). Each novice therapist will have unique strengths and challenges in skill development. As the expert, supervisors can guide the novice through developmental improvements in their skill as a therapist.

The supervisor may be seen as a source of support, but it is partly up to the novice therapist to learn, grown, and incorporate guidance. Many therapists early in training fail to appreciate that most of their anxiety comes from their own standards and expectations, not from instructors or supervisors. Only novice therapists can eliminate their own feelings of self-consciousness and doubt. It is okay to feel unsure in these early stages. However, part of the development process of the psychotherapist is to face these feelings and work to change them. By setting aside concerns about being evaluated, the novice therapist can attend to being completely focused and fully present with the client. Faculty members have a job to make sure that all students get through the graduate program, move on to internship, and get employed in the field. Therefore, faculty members are motivated to help and provide feedback that guides the student toward improvement, even when it might be interpreted as criticism. Over time, the novice therapist gets comfortable with the basics of being responsible for their clients and begins to form a layer of technical skills, knowledge of interventions, and successful therapeutic experiences. As this cocoon forms, new influences arise and must be incorporated into the novice therapist's skill set.

## Integrating Evidence-Based Practice with Common Skills

As novice therapists continue to build skills and grow in confidence, they are learning to integrate various sources of education, research, and experience. In this stage of development, the chrysalis is growing thick as the novice therapist "consumes" more readings and experiences. The novice therapist must confront several seemingly black-and-white debates: Are you a researcher or are you a clinician? Do you abide with cognitive behavioral theories or psychodynamic therapy? How much do you feel that therapy is useful because of common factors or treatment-specific techniques? These questions may begin during interviews for graduate school, and continue until the trainee realizes there is an acceptable middle ground between the two extremes.

One professional debate that arises early for the novice therapist as they integrate classroom learning with experiential practicums is that of the common factors of therapy versus treatment-specific interventions. While advancing through graduate school coursework and attending a range of clinical placement sites, novice therapists are typically taught the way in which therapy is done at that respective institution. Beneficially, through interactions with supervisors and professors with different backgrounds trainees can gain knowledge of various ways to engage in therapy. However, in the process of learning how to be a therapist, how to document, and how to hold discussions with peers and superiors about the therapeutic interaction, it can feel as though you have to learn a new language.

Specific treatments like cognitive behavioral therapy, behavioral activation, exposure and response prevention, and others have prescribed techniques and methods. Common factors are generally defined as therapeutic variables that are seen across different interventions, but are not specific to a particular technique or theory (Stamoulos et al. 2016). One definition of common therapeutic factors includes: the supportive bond between therapist and client, a healing setting, an explanation for emotional distress based on psychological and cultural information, an explanation that is acceptable to the client and flexible to individual needs, and change that is positive, helpful, or adaptive in some way (Laska, Gurman, and Wampold 2014). These nonspecific factors emphasize the importance of rapport with the client and adequate explanation of reasons for choice of intervention. Experienced psychotherapists reported patient engagement, affective experiencing, and therapeutic alliance to be among the most important common factors to be implemented for beneficial treatment outcomes (Tschacher, Junghan, and Pfammatter 2014, Stamoulos et al. 2016). Remembering the core common factors can be a great way for novice therapists to feel confident in therapy, even when they are still learning specific interventions.

Acknowledgment of the common factors that are present in psychotherapy is not an attempt to replace more evidence-based treatments. There is no such thing as a common factor treatment and one of the common factors includes properly describing a particular disorder and related symptoms, as well as explaining the treatment modality chosen to target these problems (Laska and Wampold 2014). The common factors are meant to be flexible and adapted to individual clients in the broader context of therapy (Laska and Wampold 2014). Therefore, relying on nonspecific factors does not negate the use of specific evidence-based treatments. As a novice therapist, there is tangible pressure to follow the intervention or orientation most often espoused by the graduate program or clinical placement. However, it can be helpful to remember that a lot is accomplished in therapy outside of the particular intervention.

The importance of using evidence-based treatments is not to be overlooked. Staying up to date with properly researched and empirically supported therapeutic interventions is vital. Yet, the issue is more complex than reading journal articles and published treatment manuals in the search for a recipe for effective therapy. Evidence-based practice necessarily includes empirically supported treatments, but is not made up of these treatments alone (Laska, Gurman, and Wampold 2014). In a comparison study looking at cognitive behavioral therapies versus common factors, rapport was shown to have the strongest relationship with a subsequent decrease in depressive symptoms (Antunes-Alves et al. 2018). It is not helpful to become focused on providing therapy according to published guidelines or manuals and strictly adhering to a particular approach. Flexibility is an important part of being a therapist at any level of expertise (Kendall and Frank 2018). For a novice therapist, it can feel challenging to juggle general ideas from a common factors approach alongside guidelines in a published treatment manual.

When looking to meta-analytic work, the evidence seems conflicted regarding whether specific treatment factors or broad contextual models of common factors are more effective (Marcus et al. 2014). In fact, common and specific factors have been shown to be correlated to each other throughout therapy, suggesting less of a dichotomy than is often portrayed (de Felice et al. 2019). Novice therapists may notice their supervisor has a strong allegiance to a particular therapeutic orientation, especially when debating the mechanisms of effective treatment. At this stage of training, it may be important for the novice to listen to the reasons why another therapist feels strongly about a particular approach.

The ongoing debate in favor of common factor elements of therapy suggests that proponents of evidence-based treatments overemphasize differences between treatments while omitting aspects, such as the therapeutic alliance or the subjective experience of the client, that are related to beneficial outcomes (Wampold and Bhati 2004). Much overlap exists between the arguments for common versus specific factors of therapy, with therapists on both sides agreeing that there are cross-modal and intervention-specific aspects present in most treatments as well as agreeing about the importance of treatment based in research evidence (Mulder, Murray, and Rucklidge 2017). In order to become a skilled clinician, the novice therapist is advised to focus on learning many languages of therapy rather siding with one particular theory. In most situations, it is best to appreciate the many layers of the psychotherapy process. Thus, common factors provide a subtle but essential background layer, important in every session but usually working unnoticed by therapist or client. In contrast, specific treatment techniques serve as a prominent foreground image, highly visible to both therapist and client. Together, these two layers set the stage for an effective therapy session.

Factors relating to the clients or the therapists play an important role in how therapy unfolds. Any standardized intervention will look different depending on client factors. Patient-related variables, such as distress, impairment, and coping style have been shown to have a significant effect on therapeutic outcome independent of treatment factors and the therapeutic alliance (Beutler et al. 2012). Age race, gender, marital status, sexual orientation, socioeconomic class and other identities impact various treatment outcomes in therapy and emphasize a need for cultural competency (Sue and Lam 2002). Therapist factors can play a role in the process and outcome of psychotherapy sessions. In general, being more active and less passive may be more effective in short-term therapy, while being more genial and less forceful may result in better treatment outcomes in long-term therapy (Heinonen et al. 2012). Just as clients may be more or less suited to particular interventions, therapists may vary in their delivery of those interventions. Novice therapists can pay attention to their own personality qualities and interpersonal style to appreciate how these factors can have an impact on the effectiveness of treatment across contexts.

Clients may have their own perspective on the debate between standardized therapy and common factors. A sample of 329 adults from the United States showed a significant preference for seeking therapy focusing on common factors over therapy emphasizing specific evidence-based treatments (Swan and Heesacker 2013). What is deemed best from the client perspective can vary as well. The same therapeutic techniques that were identified as helpful in one context were noted to be a hindrance in another (Swift, Tompkins, and Parkin 2017). Rarely does a client have enough background to come into therapy knowing the type of intervention that best meets their symptom profile. It is up to therapists to navigate among various manualized interventions, particular theoretical orientations, and various common factors that help to relieve client distress. Adults receiving therapy through a psychology training clinic reported benefit from both treatment-specific factors, such as skills training, insight, and emotional processing, and common factors, such as non-judgmental listening and empathy (Swift, Tompkins, and Parkin 2017). The specific or common factors debate is moot. It is more helpful for a novice therapist to focus on the client's problems, needs, and what is best for them as an individual.

Therapeutic change occurs on a number of levels. First-order change refers to the result of applying therapeutic techniques directly to a symptom or problem, aiming for a straight-forward reduction of symptom severity. In contrast, second-order change refers to the results seen in the broader context in which the symptoms or problems tend to occur (Brown 2015). The most effective evidence-based treatment includes a focus on four components: the cognitive and emotional processes, the common factors of therapy, first-order and second-order change, and the principles present in disorder-specific therapeutic techniques (Brown 2015). Both treatment-specific methods and common factors have their use in effective therapy. Common factors in therapy may alert the therapist to central therapeutic issues and thus serve to organize various therapeutic principles in the context of therapy (Oddli, Nissen-Lie, and Halvorsen 2016).

Consuming a foundation of knowledge about these aspects and remaining active in determining what works best will help novice therapists grow and remain flexible in developing therapeutic skills.

As a novice therapist, it is important to focus on learning and improving skills. Being sidetracked by having to choose a side in the many debates surrounding the identity of psychologists can distract from this goal and lead to a sense of not knowing what to do in therapy. In developing as a therapist, it is important to start with who you are as a person, build your own style of relating to clients, and then hone in on disorders, age groups, and therapy techniques that align with who you are as a person. In many ways, therapists learn more from their clients than from any classroom course or supervision relationship. Ongoing clinical experience for therapists throughout their career path is essential whether one remains mostly a clinician, serves as faculty, or works in research (Overholser 2019). The best learning happens by doing, and from an early stage therapists grow through learning directly from clients, what works in practice, and what the therapy process is like firsthand.

Psychologists in training face a number of decision points. As novice therapists, it can feel overwhelming to decide what type of psychologist one plans to become with definitive confidence. In many ways learning never stops, and whether a novice aligns more with the common factors or treatment-specific techniques may change throughout their career and depend on the typical client population being treated. Remember to not take the chrysalis stage of becoming a butterfly for granted. Faculty and mentors can serve as resources and guides, but do not require mimicking or imitation. Novice therapists can take the skills learned in training, science, and knowledge of human behavior, and put them toward interpretation of psychological trends and theoretical orientations. Using the huge amount of information available to determine where the therapeutic allegiance lies will take time, and being open to disagreement, change, and shifts will help in the long run when creating a therapeutic identity. Navigating persistent debates within the field of psychology provides opportunities to engage in metamorphosis and growth.

## DEVELOPING A THERAPEUTIC ORIENTATION AND PROFESSIONAL IDENTITY

Development of a therapeutic orientation and professional identity as a therapist is a creative, individualized, and nuanced process. Some novice therapists might know with certainty early on how they identify as a therapist. Others may make small adjustments to their identity throughout their graduate training and across their career. It is important find the therapeutic orientation that fits the person's professional training, clinical experience, and worldview (Laska and Wampold 2014). Developing a therapeutic orientation may be different for everyone, but this process consistently overlaps with the therapist's personal belief system. Similar to a butterfly beginning to take shape within their cocoon, novice therapists develop their professional identity within the safe confines of supervised clinical experience. It may be best to view this as a long-term process of professional growth with many twists and turns.

The primary traditions of therapeutic orientation are psychoanalytic/ psychodynamic, behavioral, cognitive, humanistic/existential/ experiential, and integrative/ eclectic/ holistic (APA 2009). Personality factors are associated with therapist identification as humanistic, psychodynamic, or cognitive-behavioral (Boswell, Castonguay, and Pincus 2009). The training program, personal history, clinical supervisors, and peers also influence the novice therapist's opinions and perspectives about the optimal type of psychotherapy. To a novice therapist, it may appear that others have already established a clearly defined style and orientation for therapy. However, most mental health professionals adjust their theoretical orientation and style of therapy over time based on a variety of influences.

Graduate training is not broad enough to cover all psychotherapy orientations. Thus, teasing apart why certain individuals choose a specific approach is complicated by their access to training opportunities. There may be a certain extent of socialization that occurs as a trainee begins to adjust their philosophy to that of their training program (Wolff and Auckenthaler 2014). During the early stages of training, certain orientations may be preferred over others. One study of master's level psychologists found that those with a cognitive behavioral orientation reported prioritizing a strong foundation of scientific evidence, official recognition of the method, and financial security in choosing an orientation, while those with a psychodynamic orientation reported prioritizing the role of personal experiences and life history background (Safi et al. 2017). As training continues, there is an ongoing process of adjustment based on experience being an actual therapist. Among psychotherapy trainees who were learning about cognitive behavioral therapy, participants reported using assimilation of new experiences and reorganization of existing definitions in a constantly adapting version of their theoretical orientation (Wolff and Auckenthaler 2014). It is one thing to read about a therapy, or even to become trained in it, but it is another to accumulate experience with how it is actually applied with different clients and assorted diagnoses.

The process of uncovering a therapeutic orientation and establishing one's professional identity is similar to the restructuring that occurs inside the larva before the butterfly emerges. A long process of reorganizing one's opinions, personal values, scientific knowledge, and therapy skills inevitably involves a mix of personal and professional parts of oneself. Cultivation of a therapeutic orientation and identity involves a personal core and a professional extension, defined by ongoing refinement of personal qualities alongside the adoption of new skills, techniques, and theories (Maruniakova, Rihacek, and Roubal 2017). In many careers, there is a clear distinction between a personal and a professional role. In the world of therapy, psychologists often need to integrate their personal and professional identities to form a stable persona across contexts. Within a therapy session, self-disclosure can be used to show understanding and empathy toward a client. Sharing a personal experience similar to that of a client can assist novice therapists in modelling healthy coping skills in the client, even when the specific experience is not shared through self-disclosure. For example, therapists having gone through the grief stages themselves may increase the ability to empathize with a grieving client, even if that specific experience is not disclosed by the therapist.

Additionally, the integration of personal and professional identities is crucial to healthy processing of the emotional content that is often discussed in therapy sessions.

Some novice therapists identify with a division between a true self and a false self, with the false persona serving as a protection against vulnerability and insult (Eckler-Hart 1987). In training, teasing the personal and professional selves apart is a challenge and therefore possibly more intimidating. Evaluation as a therapist can be interpreted as evaluation as a person (Eckler-Hart 1987). Acknowledging the presence of the person in the profession can help to improve insight while a professional identity is forming. There can be significant overlap between how therapists interact in close personal relationships and how their identified theoretical orientation recommends interacting with clients in therapy (Heinonen and Orlinsky 2013). As a novice therapist, understanding the nuanced overlap between personal and professional lives is particularly challenging because the two roles seem to blend together. Novice therapists may learn about the ethical implications of behaving irresponsibly with clients. However, errors made in therapy, such as mistakenly offending a client, can provide opportunities to show that therapists are human and model how to handle such errors.

For novice therapists, acknowledging the blend of personal and professional selves can be an important step in professional development. In one model of personal and professional development, Sheikh et. al (2007) identified reflection as a central learning component for therapists in training, facilitated by clear roles of personal self-awareness in the professional realm, establishment of learning goals related to personal and professional functioning, and effective use of support systems. Having an understanding of personal development helps novice therapists grow in a way similar to how clients grow in therapy. Personal development as a therapist involves strengthening natural abilities, allowing room for personal values in therapy, learning limits, using personal experience appropriately, and controlling subjective reactions in session (Maruniakova, Rihacek, and Roubal 2017). With experience, this awareness and sensitivity may naturally mature. As a novice grows comfortable in the role of therapist, it becomes easier to bring more of their personal self into the therapeutic work (Salter and Rhodes 2018).

An integrative therapist utilizes a range of interventions in their practice and incorporates ideas from a variety of theories as needed for diverse clinical circumstances. Therapists may overestimate the degree to which they abide by a specific therapeutic orientation, with a greater number of therapists reporting eclectic attitudes and practices (Sandell et al. 2006). Most therapists are trained under a certain orientation, but integrate a new identity through postgraduate experiences (Boswell, Castonguay, and Pincus 2009). Novice therapists may find comfort in identifying with a particular therapeutic orientation because of the structure and direction it provides. Questioning and broadening of this orientation may happen later. As therapists become more autonomous, they may simultaneously become more integrated in their therapeutic orientation, based on qualities like congruence between a specific model and a therapist's preferences as well as perceived efficacy of a specific model in everyday practice (Rihacek, Danelova, and Cermak 2012).

Therapists who identify as integrationist may go through multiple stages to arrive at their eventual therapeutic orientation and professional identity. Based on psychotherapist autobiographies, Rihacek and Danelova (2016) described a three-stage developmental model including the adherence phase, the destabilization phase, and the consolidation phase. Adherence was categorized by identifying with a particular theoretical orientation, destabilization by starting to explore other approaches while weakening the original orientation based on increased experience, and consolidation by development of a more flexible and heterogeneous integrated system (Rihacek and Danelova 2016). Likely, identifying these stages and the steps toward becoming an integrationist is difficult without the use of hindsight. However, being aware of these potential transitions, as well as the ways in which therapists change, could help the novice therapist assign less importance to certainty around their early therapeutic identity.

Self-awareness plays a central role in general development of the novice therapist. Transformative learning is central to the development of a professional identity and is defined as an expanding awareness through critical examination and reflection of beliefs, values, and underlying assumptions (Dong et al. 2018). Practicing being present in the here and now of therapy could assist in growth and prosperity as a therapist. Mindfulness and acceptance may be useful to help novice therapists make the number of transitions involved in professional development including idealism to realism, burnout to rejuvenation, compartmentalization to integration, and external to internal validation (Dong et al. 2018). Additionally, with more experience and advancement in a career as a therapist, openness to reflection on one's own emotions, thoughts, and values increases, a process noted to be essential to maintaining appropriate boundaries (Salter and Rhodes 2018). Not everyone knows what kind of therapist they will be every step along the way to expertise. Openness to this uncertainty will help the novice therapist manage the stress of developing through the different stages.

A shift in self-confidence impacts alignment with a particular orientation. Therapists learning cognitive behavioral therapy may develop professional confidence gradually, moving from externally-based confidence in the treatment based on reading published research, to having internalized confidence in the treatment based on prior successful clinical experience, and finally to having self-confidence as a therapist based on years of training, education and accumulated clinical experience (Maruniakova and Rihacek 2018). In this model, externally-based confidence comes from knowledge of cognitive behavioral therapy, internalized confidence comes from positive experiences using this intervention, and self-confidence comes from understanding the limits of cognitive behavioral therapy and actively searching for other types of treatment and personal resources (Maruniakova and Rihacek 2018). Having confidence as a therapist means both having confidence in yourself and your abilities as well as in the therapeutic intervention being used. As novice therapists move forward, therapeutic identity grows stronger through several developmental milestones, progressing toward pre-doctoral internship, post-doctoral fellowship, and eventually an independent career.

Aspects of personal development may be overlooked in some clinical psychology training programs, with all attention dedicated to the development of professional skills (Salter and Rhodes 2018). Supervisors and faculty members could devote more attention to graduate student personal development within the professional realm. Often the novice therapist may feel overwhelmed by the available options and pushed to feel a particular way by the training program or by peers who already advocate for strong theoretical orientation preferences. Faculty mentors can offer a more mature perspective, helping novice therapists realize that they have a whole career before them to learn the language of therapy, and develop their own theoretical orientation. Occasionally, when juggling the development of personal and professional selves, training gets off track or a therapy session feels disjointed. These are important times for faculty members, mentors, and clinical supervisors to remember their own wayward path through the maze of professional development.

Novice therapists can feel overwhelmed by their own personal expectations to learn, decipher, test, practice, choose, and believe a spectrum of therapies and psychological information. Psychotherapy is a complex task. Professional development takes into account the robust number of interventions, the numerous conflicting opinions of professionals, and an abundance of mixed meta-analytic findings in the field. There may be an emotional toll on the therapist resulting from managing these various aspects of being an ethical practicing psychotherapist (Rodríguez 2018). The overlap between the personal self and the professional self helps a novice therapist work through the early stages of developing a theoretical orientation and professional identity. All therapists can remind themselves of what brought them into the field and what it means to relate to a client on a personal level. Skills and theoretical orientation develop with experience. Additionally, an acknowledgement of the option of integration across orientations and identities opens up a whole world of possibilities. Integrative therapy means conducting evidence-based practice and methods without having to identify myopically with any one theory. During earlier stages of training, it is important for novice therapists to remember that they do not need to have all the answers regarding their professional identity.

## CONTINUING THE PROFESSIONAL EVOLUTION

There is a lot more to being a therapist than just completing the specific procedures of an intervention. As a novice therapist, trying to learn as much as possible while putting that knowledge into practice can be intimidating. In the early stages of being a psychotherapist, there appears to be a heavy focus on professional and skill development. An important aspect of being a therapist, whether a novice or an expert, is the ability to self-reflect and to balance personal belief systems with evidence-based practice. In a study that interviewed psychologists who had been praised for clinical wisdom throughout their career, Levitt and Piazza-Bonin (2016) highlighted the core messages relayed to those early in their career. Therapists must go beyond basic intelligence to foster emotional intelligence, social intelligence, and knowledge about the self (Levitt and Piazza-Bonin 2016). Vulnerability and ambiguity, the ability to be wrong, to not know the answers, and to change course are indispensable for therapeutic wisdom (Levitt and Piazza-Bonin 2016). Not getting stuck on a pre-established way therapy must unfold is vital to attuning treatment to the individual and applying interventions to different contexts (Levitt and Piazza-Bonin 2016).

As a novice therapist, it is enticing to think about a time in the future when all skills have been mastered and all clients have been figured out. However, becoming a therapist means that there will always be more knowledge to acquire, more questions to ask, and more problems to solve. Once a novice therapist obtains a doctoral degree, the journey of professional development is not finished. Believing that one has the answers to everything is a quick route towards professional decline. For example, there is evidence that professional psychologists become less effective with their clients over time (Goldberg et al. 2016). This can be attributed to a phenomenon called "therapist drift," in which therapists fail to deliver optimal evidence-based psychotherapy despite having the knowledge and skills to do so (Waller and Turner 2016). Therapist drift may occur when expert therapists believe they already know everything, and subsequently fail to actively learn and improve in their craft. As a professional therapist, it is important to admit when one does not know the answer and to always be hungry for knowledge. The research literature will continue to expand, new therapeutic techniques will be created, and the psychological field will grow and diversify. It is the job of a therapist to acknowledge these truths, as a large part of being an expert is recognizing and adapting to change. A good example of the psychological field changing is the recent integration of telehealth and psychotherapy. The novice therapists of fifty years ago most likely never anticipated that they would be conducting psychotherapy through video conferencing at some point in their careers. However, as the field changes, therapists are able to learn and adapt in order to continue providing care for their clients. It is important that as novice therapists become experts over the span of their careers, that they remain both humble and eager to grow and improve in their profession.

The formation of an eventual butterfly takes time, and the style and values of a psychotherapist may continue to evolve over the course of their career, as they develop skills in different domains and change theoretical orientations based on experience. While the focus here is on that of the novice therapist navigating early clinical training and work in graduate school, the developmental processes continue through internship, post-doctoral fellowship, early years as a Ph.D., and later years as an expert. Professional development as a therapist includes personal domains, such as life philosophy, personality, previous experiences, and professional domains, such as graduate training, clients, and professional development (Bitar, Bean, and Bermúdez 2007). Professional development comes with a number of different experiences including adopting rules and ethical codes, digesting new information, increased clinical experience, and incorporation of natural tendencies (Maruniakova, Rihacek, and Roubal 2017). Opportunities for these various influences shift as the transition is made through stages like internship and beyond. New locations, training sites, supervisors, populations, and teaching opportunities all force a young psychologist to speak for what they believe in and defend their own professional values, forming a firm foundation by testing the ideas in a public forum. Ongoing professional activity as a therapist is essential for forming a solid professional identity. Clinical psychologists who shift into academic or administrative careers alone are left with a faded memory of clinical contact that usually lacks substance. Keeping up with all aspects of therapeutic identity is important for creating the fundamental structure on which to stand as a therapist.

## CONCLUSION

The transition from a caterpillar to a butterfly involves a great deal of consumption, growth, rearranging, and development. Similarly, for novice therapists, there is a long road of metamorphosis ahead. There exists the more obvious and defined track from research assistant to graduate student to intern to post-doc to career psychologist. However, underlying this path are stages of growth and change that are more subtle in nature. These stages include working through the nervous anticipation of being with a client for the first time, learning how to be comfortable and capable when conducting therapy, grappling with ongoing debates in the field about which intervention is most effective, and integrating knowledge and experience across the lifetime into a coherent therapeutic identity.

Professional identity development is a process that begins in graduate school and continues across the entire professional career (Dong et al. 2018). As a novice therapist, it is easy to convince yourself that you will never be as good as the seasoned therapists with whom you interact. You will never know everything. To a certain extent, the exact mechanisms and aspects of psychotherapy that are effective remain unknown. Chaos theory, when applied to psychotherapeutic processes, has been shown to be a useful computational model of prediction (Schiepek et al. 2017). This is not hopeless, but is hopeful, in that there is progress to be made and we each contribute to that progress in new and creative ways. Development as a psychologist, from caterpillar to butterfly, must involve internal and external change. There appears broadly to be a balance between growth and depletion, as well as healing and stress, that underlie the process of professional development (Rønnestad et al. 2018). There are ups and downs to becoming a clinical psychologist, and the trajectory for every therapist looks different, just as every client's journey through therapy varies. In a study of psychotherapists across the lifespan, work and life satisfaction were shown to significantly increase with age, while depletion significantly decreased with age (Orlinsky and Rønnestad 2015). Above all, novice therapists should remember that it gets better. Young trainees should take advantage of the amazing stage of learning where they are able to begin, fresh and open to each new moment. The novice therapists of today will be late-career psychologists of tomorrow, helping those earlier in training feel comfortable in their roles.

To novice therapists, graduate students, faculty, mentors, and supervisors alike, take away from this chapter that we all journey through these stages and do so in unique ways. For some, the end goals are obvious from the beginning, and for others, they change with each new clinical interaction. Remind yourself of the normality of progress paired with mistakes, of strong beliefs paired with changed perspectives, and of experience or wisdom paired with novelty or new viewpoints. These are the aspects that make the process of training in clinical psychology so unique, enticing, and intellectually challenging. The simultaneous common and varied stages of development from caterpillar to butterfly are what unite us as a field and what allow us to help clients grow.

## References

Adebiyi, Munirat Olayinka, Samuel Kolawole Mosaku, Omolola Oladunni Irinoye, and Oyeyemi Olajumoke Oyelade. 2018. "Socio-demographic and clinical factors associated with relapse in mental illness." *International journal of Africa nursing sciences* 8:149-153.

Antunes-Alves, Sara, Boris Vukovic, Marina Milyavskaya, Ueli Kramer, Keith Dobson, and Martin Drapeau. 2018. "Therapist interventions and patient outcome: addressing the common versus specific factor debate." *Archives of Psychiatry and Psychotherapy* 20 (3):7-25.

APA. 2009. "*Different approaches to psychotherapy*." accessed August 25. https://www.apa.org/topics/therapy/psychotherapy-approaches.

Beutler, Larry E, Bryan Forrester, Delores Gallagher-Thompson, Larry Thompson, and Joseph B Tomlins. 2012. "Common, specific, and treatment fit variables in psychotherapy outcome." *Journal of Psychotherapy Integration* 22 (3):255.

Bitar, George W, Roy A Bean, and J Maria Bermúdez. 2007. "Influences and processes in theoretical orientation development: A grounded theory pilot study." *The American Journal of Family Therapy* 35 (2):109-121.

Boswell, James F, Louis G Castonguay, and Aaron L Pincus. 2009. "Trainee theoretical orientation: Profiles and potential predictors." *Journal of Psychotherapy integration* 19 (3):291.

Brown, Jac. 2015. "Specific techniques vs. common factors? Psychotherapy integration and its role in ethical practice." *American Journal of Psychotherapy* 69 (3):301-316.

Coppock, Timothy E, Jesse J Owen, Elena Zagarskas, and Melissa Schmidt. 2010. "The relationship between therapist and client hope with therapy outcomes." *Psychotherapy Research* 20 (6):619-626.

Cynkar, Amy, and Dana Schwartz. 2007. "Facing your first clients." *gradPSYCH Magazine*.

de Felice, Giulio, Alessandro Giuliani, Sibel Halfon, Silvia Andreassi, Giulia Paoloni, and Franco Orsucci. 2019. "The misleading Dodo Bird verdict. How much of the outcome variance is explained by common and specific factors?" *New Ideas in Psychology* 54. doi: 10.1016/j.newideapsych.2019.01.006.

Dong, ShengLi, Linda Miles, Neil Abell, and Jadelyn Martinez. 2018. "Development of professional identity for counseling professionals: A mindfulness-based perspective." *International Journal for the Advancement of Counselling* 40 (4):469-480.

Dowell, Nia M, and Jeffrey S Berman. 2013. "Therapist nonverbal behavior and perceptions of empathy, alliance, and treatment credibility." *Journal of Psychotherapy Integration* 23 (2):158.

Duff, Carlton T, and Robinder P Bedi. 2010. "Counsellor behaviours that predict therapeutic alliance: From the client's perspective." *Counselling psychology quarterly* 23 (1):91-110.

Eckler-Hart, Anton H. 1987. "True and false self in the development of the psychotherapist." *Psychotherapy: Theory, Research, Practice, Training* 24 (4):683.

Elliott, Robert, Arthur C Bohart, Jeanne C Watson, and David Murphy. 2018. "Therapist empathy and client outcome: An updated meta-analysis." *Psychotherapy* 55 (4):399.

Ellis, Thomas E. 2004. "Collaboration and a self-help orientation in therapy with suicidal clients." *Journal of Contemporary Psychotherapy* 34 (1):41-57.

Goldberg, Simon B, Tony Rousmaniere, Scott D Miller, Jason Whipple, Stevan Lars Nielsen, William T Hoyt, and Bruce E Wampold. 2016. "Do psychotherapists improve with time and experience? A longitudinal analysis of outcomes in a clinical setting." *Journal of Counseling Psychology* 63 (1):1.

Heinonen, Erkki, Olavi Lindfors, Maarit A Laaksonen, and Paul Knekt. 2012. "Therapists' professional and personal characteristics as predictors of outcome in short-and long-term psychotherapy." *Journal of Affective Disorders* 138 (3):301-312.

Heinonen, Erkki, and David Elliot Orlinsky. 2013. "Psychotherapists' personal identities, theoretical orientations, and professional relationships: Elective affinity and role adjustment as modes of congruence." *Psychotherapy Research* 23 (6):718-731.

Hill, Clara E, Jessica Stahl, and Melissa Roffman. 2007. "Training novice psychotherapists: Helping skills and beyond." *Psychotherapy: Theory, Research, Practice, Training* 44 (4):364.

Hiltunen, Arto J, Elo Kocys, and Renée Perrin-Wallqvist. 2013. "Effectiveness of cognitive behavioral therapy: An evaluation of therapies provided by trainees at a university psychotherapy training center." *PsyCh Journal* 2 (2):101-112.

Irving, Lori M, CR Snyder, Jen Cheavens, Lorraine Gravel, Julie Hanke, Pamela Hilberg, and Nicole Nelson. 2004. "The relationships between hope and outcomes at the pretreatment, beginning, and later phases of psychotherapy." *Journal of Psychotherapy Integration* 14 (4):419.

Jobes, David A, and Alan L Berman. 1993. "Suicide and malpractice liability: Assessing and revising policies, procedures, and practice in outpatient settings." *Professional Psychology: Research and Practice* 24 (1):91.

Kendall, Philip C, and Hannah E Frank. 2018. "Implementing evidence-based treatment protocols: Flexibility within fidelity." *Clinical Psychology: Science and Practice* 25 (4):e12271.

Keyes, Corey. 2007. "Towards a mentally flourishing society: Mental health promotion, not cure." *Journal of Public Mental Health* 6 (2):4.

Larsen, Denise, Wendy Edey, and Lenora Lemay. 2007. "Understanding the role of hope in counselling: Exploring the intentional uses of hope." *Counselling Psychology Quarterly* 20 (4):401-416.

Laska, Kevin M, Alan S Gurman, and Bruce E Wampold. 2014. "Expanding the lens of evidence-based practice in psychotherapy: A common factors perspective." *Psychotherapy* 51 (4):467.

Laska, Kevin M, and Bruce E. Wampold. 2014. "Ten things to remember about common factor theory." *Psychotherapy* 51 (4):519-524. doi: 10.1037/a0038245.

Lavik, Kristina O, Helga Frøysa, Karen F Brattebø, John McLeod, and Christian Moltu. 2018. "The first sessions of psychotherapy: A qualitative meta-analysis of alliance formation processes." *Journal of Psychotherapy Integration* 28 (3):348.

Levitt, Heidi M, and Elizabeth Piazza-Bonin. 2016. "Wisdom and psychotherapy: Studying expert therapists' clinical wisdom to explicate common processes." *Psychotherapy Research* 26 (1):31-47.

Mahoney, Michael J. 1997. "Psychotherapists' personal problems and self-care patterns." *Professional Psychology: Research and Practice* 28 (1):14-16. doi: 10.1037/0735-7028.28.1.14.

Marcus, David K, Debra O'Connell, Alyssa L Norris, and Abere Sawaqdeh. 2014. "Is the Dodo bird endang[illegible] 21st century? A meta-analysis of treatment comparison stu[illegible] *[illegible]ychology Review* 34 (7):519-530.

Maruniakova, Lenka, and Tomas Rihacek. 201[illegible] cognitive behavioural therapists develop professio[illegible] *Cognitive Behaviour Therapist* 11.

Maruniakova, Lenka, Tomas Rihacek, and Jan Roubal. 2[illegible] beginning counselors learn: The interaction of perso[illegible] professional experiences in counselors with an experi[illegible] orientation." *Counselling Psychology Quarterly* 30 (1):48-66.

Mulder, Roger, Greg Murray, and Julia Rucklidge. 2017. "Common versus specific factors in psychotherapy: opening the black box." *The Lancet Psychiatry* 4 (12):953-962.

Nutt Williams, Elizabeth. 2008. "A psychotherapy researcher's perspective on therapist self-awareness and self-focused attention after a decade of research." *Psychotherapy research* 18 (2):139-146.

Oddli, Hanne Weie, Helene A Nissen-Lie, and Margrethe Seeger Halvorsen. 2016. "Common therapeutic change principles as "sensitizing concepts": A key perspective in psychotherapy integration and clinical research." *Journal of Psychotherapy Integration* 26 (2):160.

Orlinsky, David E, and Michael Helge Rønnestad. 2015. "Psychotherapists growing older: A study of senior practitioners." *Journal of Clinical Psychology* 71 (11):1128-1138.

Overholser, James C. 2004. "The four pillars of psychotherapy supervision." *The Clinical Supervisor* 23 (1):1-13.

Overholser, James C. 2019. "Graduate training in psychotherapy: The importance of ongoing clinical activity for the training faculty." *Counselling and Psychotherapy Research* 19 (3):264-273.

Richardson, Clarissa ME, Wilson T Trusty, and Kylie A George. 2020. "Trainee wellness: self-critical perfectionism, self-compassion, depression, and burnout among doctoral trainees in psychology." *Counselling Psychology Quarterly* 33 (2):187-198.

Rihacek, Tomas, and Ester Danelova. 2016. "The journey of an integrationist: A grounded theory analysis." *Psychotherapy* 53 (1):78.

Rihacek, Tomas, Ester Danelova, and Ivo Cermak. 2012. "Psychotherapist development: Integration as a way to autonomy." *Psychotherapy Research* 22 (5):556-569.

Rihacek, Tomas, and Jan Roubal. 2018. "Common principles of psychotherapeutic change: Patterns of use." *British Journal of Guidance & Counselling*:1-11.

Rodríguez, Antonio Galán. 2018. "Struggling with psychological treatments comparation: Looking for practitioner's survival." *Papeles del Psicólogo* 39 (1):13-21.

Rogers, Carl R. 1957. "The necessary and sufficient conditions of therapeutic personality change." *Journal of Consulting Psychology* 21 (2):95.

Rønnestad, Michael Helge, David Orlinsky, Thomas Schroder, Thomas Skovholt, and Ulrike Willutzki. 2018. "The Professional development of counsellor and psychotherapists: Implications of empirical studies for supervision, training and practice." *Counselling and Psychotherapy Research*. doi: 10.1002/capr.12198.

Rummell, Christina M. 2015. "An exploratory study of psychology graduate student workload, health, and program satisfaction." *Professional Psychology: Research and Practice* 46 (6):391-399. doi: 10.1037/pro0000056.

Safi, Annette, Hinrich Bents, Ulrike Dinger, Johannes C Ehrenthal, Kristina Ackel-Eisnach, Wolfgang Herzog, Henning Schauenburg, and Christoph Nikendei. 2017. "Psychotherapy training: A comparative qualitative study on motivational factors and personal background of psychodynamic and cognitive behavioural psychotherapy candidates." *Journal of Psychotherapy Integration* 27 (2):186.

Salter, Marine, and Paul Rhodes. 2018. "On becoming a therapist: A narrative inquiry of personal–professional development and the training of clinical psychologists." *Australian Psychologist* 53 (6):486-492. doi: 10.1111/ap.12344.

Sandell, Rolf, Jan Carlsson, Johan Schubert, Jeanette Broberg, Anna Lazar, and Johan Grant. 2006. "Therapist attitudes and patient outcomes: I. Development and validation of the Therapeutic Attitudes Scales (TASC-2)." *Psychotherapy Research.*

Schiepek, Günter K, Kathrin Viol, Wolfgang Aichhorn, Marc-Thorsten Hütt, Katharina Sungler, David Pincus, and Helmut J Schöller. 2017. "Psychotherapy is chaotic—(Not only) in a computational world." *Frontiers in Psychology* 8:379.

Sheikh, Alia I, Derek L Milne, and Bryony V MacGregor. 2007. "A model of personal professional development in the systematic training of clinical psychologists." *Clinical Psychology & Psychotherapy: An International Journal of Theory & Practice* 14 (4):278-287.

Simpson, Skip, and Michael Stacy. 2004. "Avoiding the malpractice snare: Documenting suicide risk assessment." *Journal of Psychiatric Practice* 10 (3):185-189.

Skovholt, Thomas M, and Michael H Rønnestad. 2003. "Struggles of the novice counselor and therapist." *Journal of Career Development* 30 (1):45-58.

Stamoulos, Constantina, Lyane Trepanier, Sophia Bourkas, Stacy Bradley, Kelly Stelmaszczyk, Deborah Schwartzman, and Martin Drapeau. 2016. "Psychologists' perceptions of the importance of common factors in psychotherapy for successful treatment outcomes." *Journal of Psychotherapy Integration* 26 (3):300.

Sue, Stanley, and Amy G. Lam. 2002. "Cultural and demographic diversity." In *Psychotherapy Relationships That Work: Therapist Contributions and Responsiveness to Patients.*, 401-421. New York, NY, US: Oxford University Press.

Swan, Lawton K, and Martin Heesacker. 2013. "Evidence of a pronounced preference for therapy guided by common factors." *Journal of Clinical Psychology* 69 (9):869-879.

Swift, Joshua K, Kelley A Tompkins, and Susannah R Parkin. 2017. "Understanding the client's perspective of helpful and hindering events in psychotherapy sessions: A micro-process approach." *Journal of Clinical Psychology* 73 (11):1543-1555.

Thériault, Anne, Nicola Gazzola, and Brian Richardson. 2009. "Feelings of incompetence in novice therapists: Consequences, coping, and correctives." *Canadian Journal of Counselling and Psychotherapy* 43 (2).

Thomas, Jeremy. 2014. *The Butterflies of Britain and Ireland.* London, United Kingdom: Bloomsbury Publishing.

Topor, David R, Christopher G AhnAllen, Elizabeth A Mulligan, and Chandlee C Dickey. 2017. "Using video recordings of psychotherapy sessions in supervision: Strategies to reduce learner anxiety." *Academic Psychiatry* 41 (1):40-43.

Truell, Rory. 2001. "The stresses of learning counselling: Six recent graduates comment on their personal experience of learning counselling and what can be done to reduce associated harm." *Counselling Psychology Quarterly* 14 (1):67-89.

Tschacher, Wolfgang, Ulrich Martin Junghan, and Mario Pfammatter. 2014. "Towards a taxonomy of common factors in psychotherapy—results of an expert survey." *Clinical Psychology & Psychotherapy* 21 (1):82-96.

Veilleux, Jennifer C. 2011. "Coping with client death: Using a case study to discuss the effects of accidental, undetermined, and suicidal deaths on therapists." *Professional Psychology: Research and Practice* 42 (3):222.

Waller, Glenn, and Hannah Turner. 2016. "Therapist drift redux: Why well-meaning clinicians fail to deliver evidence-based therapy, and how to get back on track." *Behaviour Research and Therapy* 77:129-137.

Wampold, Bruce E, and Kuldhir S Bhati. 2004. "Attending to the omissions: A historical examination of evidence-based practice movements." *Professional Psychology: Research and Practice* 35 (6):563.

Wolff, Sabine, and Anna Auckenthaler. 2014. "Processes of theoretical orientation development in CBT trainees: What internal processes do psychotherapists in training undergo as they "integrate"?" *Journal of Psychotherapy Integration* 24 (3):223.

In: Psychotherapy
Editor: Hayley Boyd
ISBN: 978-1-53618-877-6


*Chapter 3*

# Dynamic Psychotherapy: Is Time the Enemy That Proves to Be an Ally?

***Joana Proença Becker[1,*], Rui Alexandre Paixão[1], PhD and Rui Aragão Oliveira[2], PhD***

[1]University of Coimbra, Coimbra, Portugal
[2]Portuguese Psychoanalytic Society, *Lisbon, Portugal*

## Abstract

Dynamic Psychotherapy (DP) emerged with the objective of overcoming the limitations of traditional psychoanalysis, thereby responding to a broader demand of patients who seek help to cope with specific problems in a shorter period of time, and who are unable to accomplish the requirements of a psychoanalytical process. However, as a product of psychoanalysis, the focus of psychodynamic treatment models is the emotional conflicts which are caused by traumatic experiences, not focusing on symptoms alone, but on what they mean. Clinical studies have shown that patients benefit from DP, and that psychoanalysis-based psychotherapies have presented a continuous state of improvement in patients. Nevertheless, these findings are confronted

* Corresponding Author's E-mail: joanapbecker@gmail.com.

by the fact that many researchers, health professionals and patients discard these psychotherapies because they are long-term treatments, in addition to the qualification and time required for training these therapists. In view of these controversies and convergences, through a vignette-based design, in addition to a literature review, this chapter explores the nuances of the psychotherapeutic process of DP. It analyzes the role of the patient's timing to achieve the treatment goals, time as a therapist's tool to provide specific interventions and time as a continuous process of the patient's growth, which does not stop with the end of therapy. The time of DP has been considered an obstacle to the appropriate investigation of its effectiveness, placing it outside the front-line of treatments for mental disorders. Time is also a reason why patients decline DP, as they often expect to have relatively few therapy sessions, even though their therapists consider the need for longer treatment. DP has traditionally placed emphasis on insight into relationship patterns and the processing of avoided emotions. Since the therapeutic processes involve the delivery of specific emotion-focused interventions tailored to a patient's capacity to process and tolerate feelings, treatments do not have a predetermined duration. This technique aims at helping patients to enhance self-understanding, as well as gain insight into their lives and present-day problems, which may allow them not only to maintain therapeutic improvements but to continue to improve beyond the treatment.

**Keywords:** dynamic psychotherapy, psychoanalysis, therapeutic process

## INTRODUCTION

Psychoanalysis is a discipline that combines the study of neurosis and a treatment method based on its results (Freud, 1913a). Studies on the subjective experiences of psychoanalytic psychotherapeutic processes have led to a better understanding of the dynamics of mental functioning, contributing to the development not only of psychoanalytic theory, but of the clinical technique and the implementation of public health programs (Aragão Oliveira and Oliveira, 2012). However, the effectiveness of psychoanalytic psychotherapies is questioned, mainly due to the impossibility of applying certain research methods. The method of randomized controlled trial (RCT) is not applicable to long-term dynamic psychotherapy or psychoanalytical therapy, since "it is neither possible to carry out a treatment according to a manual for several years, nor to offer patients who seek treatment no therapy for several years. It is impossible to create equally credible comparison conditions over years" (Leichsenring, 2005, p. 842). Since RCTs are the are commonly used to test the efficacy of medical and psychotherapeutic interventions, their results are best seen in the scientific field (Leichsenring, Klein, and Salzer, 2014), and often considered the only way of establishing psychotherapy as evidence-based (Fonagy, 2015). The time of psychoanalytic psychotherapies, therefore, has been considered an obstacle to the proper investigation of its effectiveness, placing them outside the first line of treatments for mental disorders (Becker, Paixão, Silva, Quartilho, and Custódio, 2019). Obviously, RCTs are a statistical credible mean of verifying the effect size of therapies, presenting response rates, mean values, and correlations. However, this method "masks an important heterogeneity that is often revealed by careful scrutiny of individual investigations" (Fonagy, 2015, p. 138).

Time is also a reason why patients decline to choose psychoanalytic psychotherapies, as they often expect to have relatively few therapy sessions, even though their therapists consider the need for longer treatment (Levenson, 1995). Although short-term dynamic psychotherapy has shown evidence of treatment effects superior to controls and similar to other highly recommended therapeutic approaches, proving to be a brief and relatively cost-effective treatment (Ajilchi, Nejati, Town, Wilson, and Abbass, 2016; Chavooshi, Saberi, Tavallaie, and Sahraei, 2017; Levi, Bar-Haim, Kreiss, and Fruchter, 2015), some studies have demonstrated the value of long-term psychotherapies, mentioning that they are not only more effective than no treatment or treatment as usual, but more effective than shorter forms of dynamic psychotherapy (Fonagy, 2015; Leichsenring, 2005; Leichsenring et al., 2014).

It is worth to emphasize that, although dynamic psychotherapies are based on the premise of relieving symptoms and resolving interpersonal conflicts in a shorter time than classical psychoanalysis, these therapies are focused on unconscious processes and the meaning of symptoms. As we know, "a symptom can change or disappear even if an unconscious problem remains unchanged, thereby being replaced by a symptom with different expression" (Aragão Oliveira and Oliveira, 2012, p. 47). Thus, treatment results should not be only validated by the reduction of symptoms, but the general improvements that help patients "achieve less mental rigidity, greater intrapsychic mobility and use of less primitive mental mechanisms" (Aragão Oliveira and Oliveira, 2012, p. 51). Aiming at helping patients to enhance self-understanding, gaining insight into their lives and present-day problems, "the therapeutic process involves the delivery of specific emotion-focused interventions tailored to a patient's capacity to process and tolerate feeling," which is the reason treatments do not have a predetermined duration (Becker et al., 2019; Town, Salvadori, Falkenström, Bradley, and Hardy, 2017a, p. 11).

For the last years, we have conducted literature reviews and studies on the effectiveness of DP (Becker et al., 2019; Batista, Senra, and Aragão Oliveira, 2014; Aragão Oliveira and Oliveira, 2012; Paixão, 2006; Paixão and Nunes, 2008) to identify the specificities of this technique, as well as its obstacles and advantages. Our clinical experience has also been instrumental in verifying the benefits of DP in the treatment of several mental disorders, and delineating research in this field. DP has been shown to be an effective method in the treatment of several psychopathologies. And, despite being similar to other therapeutic approaches during treatment, this technique leads to long-term results, with patients maintaining their state of improvement after the end of their treatments (Becker et al., 2019). The findings that psychoanalysis-based psychotherapies have shown a continuous state of improvement in patients are confronted by the fact that many researchers, health professionals and patients discard these psychotherapies because they are long-term treatments, in addition to the qualification and time required for training these therapists. Although DP studies mention this perception of time as an obstacle and an advantage (Lilliengren, Johansson, Town, Kisely, and Abbass, 2017; Ness et al., 2018), this aspect is not properly explored. In view of these controversies and convergences, this chapter explores the role of time in the therapeutic process, the subjectivity of time reflected or blurred in the achievement of treatment goals. Time as an obstacle motivated us to explore the nuances of the psychotherapeutic process of DP, analyzing the role of the patient's timing to achieve the treatment goals, time as a therapist's tool to provide specific interventions and time as a continuous process of patient's growth, which does not end with the end of therapy.

This chapter followed a vignette-based design (Evans et al., 2015) while analyzing the therapeutic process of DP technique, and the variances in patient responses. A previous narrative literature review on DP (Becker et al., 2019) and studies on psychoanalytic theory have supported the description of the specificities of this technique, focusing on the role of time in the therapeutic process. This chapter derived from clinical experiences of the authors, and met methodological recommendations of Evans et al. (2015): the vignettes are no longer than necessary; they were carefully edited in order to be clear, follow a similar structure, and highlight the key aspects of interest; the authors avoided placing the patient in the vignettes; being neutral with respect to cultural and socio-economic factors.

## THEORETICAL PERSPECTIVES

Psychoanalysis is a psychological theory, a therapeutic practice, and a research method on unconscious processes developed by Sigmund Freud between 1885 and 1939, who was initially interested in understanding the hysterical phenomena. Through the treatment of his patients, Freud realized that the mind was an ever-changing system, and most of its activities took place outside consciousness. "Unconscious mental activity affects conscious thoughts, feelings, and behaviors" (Cabaniss, Cherry, Douglas, and Schwartz, 2011, p. 4). The first psychoanalytic studies and attempts to treat hysterical patients resorted to hypnosis, which was subsequently replaced by the free association method. Free association is a method aimed to be patients aware of their inner experience. Through encouraging patients to say whatever comes into their minds without editing, this method seeks to reveal associations and connections that might otherwise not go uncovered (Cabaniss et al., 2011). This method made it possible to apply psychoanalysis to more cases of hysteria, other neuroses, and even healthy people (Freud, 1913a).

Psychoanalysis, which aims to access unconscious elements to find a solution to patients' symptoms, revolutionized the interaction between patient and therapist, by the frequency of the sessions, the topics addressed (childhood experiences, whishes, and fantasies), and the theory of how the mind works (Freud, 1912). Through theories about hysterical phenomena (Freud, 1893), group psychology (Freud, 1921), signal and automatic anxiety (Freud, 1926), it is possible to group knowledge that helps to understand and treat different psychopathologies. However, the psychoanalytic approaches are not in the first line of treatments, which may be a consequence of the lack of studies on its effectiveness. Freud (1912) stated that research and treatment coincide in psychoanalysis, however, the success of treatment is hindered in those cases that are previously destined to scientific research and treated according to its requirements. Freud (1912) recognized that, for scientific publication, it would be necessary to establish protocols and make notes of the sessions, which could not be prohibited. Nevertheless, he contested this procedure and stated that the correct conduct for the analyst is not to speculate during the analysis and to submit the collected material to a synthetic thinking after the analysis is completed.

In the past decades, there has been an increase in publications on psychoanalytic psychotherapies processes (Becker et al., 2019; Ness et al., 2018), including comparative studies that measure efficacy of two or more therapeutic approaches in the treatment of specific mental disorders (Chavooshi et al., 2017; Levi et al., 2015). However, these studies emphasize significant methodological shortcomings, such as limited number of samples, lack of assessment with standardized instruments, lack of control group, and difference in the duration of psychotherapies (Lilliengren et al., 2017; Perry, Bond, and Békes, 2017). In studies that use the comparative strategy, seen as beneficial for external validity, the operative aspects within the treatments are neglect (Chavooshi et al.,

2017). In a reductionist manner, there are three designs of studies adopted when researching the effectiveness of psychotherapies, and where the main object of psychoanalytic work, the unconscious, is not privileged. Experimental design studies favor the high control of variables and the determination of expected results, presenting, therefore, different conditions from those observed in clinical practice. Naturalistic studies of the psychotherapeutic process, aimed to verify the effectiveness, underline the gains obtained by patients, usually based on the assessment of symptoms. Efficiency studies aim to evaluate the therapeutic process; however, tend to focus on producing results with minimal resources and efforts (Aragão Oliveira and Oliveira, 2012). The last two ones are applicable for assessing the effectiveness of long-term treatments, even though the RCTs are the most used in psychotherapy outcome research.

Although the lack of controlled studies can be a reason to keep psychoanalytic approaches out of the first line of treatments, the frequency of sessions and duration of the treatment are also considered obstacles for patients to seek therapies derived from psychoanalysis. Freud saw his patients every day, except on Sundays and holidays, considering that less than six times a week was allowed only for mild cases or advanced treatments, which could be three hours of therapy a week. According to Freud (1913b), infrequent work can prevent the therapist from following the patient's real experiences, leading therapy to the risk of taking secondary paths. Regarding the duration of the treatment, Freud said it is almost impossible to be determined.

> To shorten analytic treatment is a justifiable wish, and its fulfilment, as we shall learn, is being attempted along various lines. Unfortunately, it is opposed by a very important factor, namely, the slowness with which deep-going changes in the mind are accomplished – in the last resort, no doubt, the 'timelessness' of our unconscious processes. (Freud, 1913b, p. 130)

Freud's position was opposite to the active technique of Ferenczi, and the development of the concept of "reciprocal analysis," which was the source of the conflict developed between them. Ferenczian theories played a fundamental role in the changes in psychoanalytic technique, mainly due to the importance assigned to the transference and the countertransference, and the role played by the analyst, who can use transferential aspects as a technical resource, aspects previously considered to be placed outside the therapeutic process. In Ferenczi's words (last notes of his Diary, written on October 2, 1932): "Once mutuality has been attempted, one-sided analysis then is no longer possible – not productive" (Conci, 2019, p. 8). Despite divergent thoughts, the constant dialogue with Freud was imperative for the development of Ferenczi's technique.

> Ferenczi experienced with Freud – as analyst, colleague and friend – the kind of "psychoanalytic home" that he was able to create for and with his patients. Indeed, the same is true for his Clinical diary, which we can reconsider in terms of Ferenczi's attempt to protect the "professional and scientific home" that he had built with Freud. (Conci, 2019, p. 9)

The active stance proposed by Ferenczi, and later defended in a jointly book that he published with Otto Rank (Ferenczi and Rank, 1925), aimed to speed up psychoanalytical process. Interested in rewarding and reinforcing patient´s associations, Ferenczi and Rank highlighted the "here-and-now" aspects of the therapeutic relationship, considering that the reconstruction of the past (childhood events) could lead to stronger intellectual defenses (Sifneos, 1979).

Ferenczi's concepts of active stance and reciprocal analysis may be considered the first movement to shorten the duration of psychoanalytic therapies and, therefore, to the development of dynamic psychotherapies. Dynamic Psychotherapy (DP) emerged with the objective of overcoming the limitations of traditional psychoanalysis, thereby responding to a broader demand of patients who seek help to cope with specific problems in a short term. Especially when symptoms provoke social and occupational impairments, patients need a short-term solution, making it essential to focus on symptoms and suffering that led them to seek the treatment (Becker et al., 2019).

Freud coined the word psychodynamics, which means "the forces of the mind that are in motion," when he realized that the mind was an ever-changing system, and most of its activities took place outside consciousness. DP is a treatment aimed at improving the mental and emotional health of a patient, considering that "the dynamic elements in the unconscious affect conscious thoughts, feelings, and behaviors" (Cabaniss et al., 2011, p. 4). The premise of this technique is to focus on patients' needs by conducting psychotherapeutic interventions to a specific goal in an agreement between patient and therapist. "The therapist is not a 'quiet sounding board' or a 'passive observer', but neither is the psychoanalyst" (Sifneos, 1979, p. 94). This premise aims at providing symptom relief and the resolution of interpersonal conflicts in a shorter time than classical Psychoanalysis (Gabbard, 2014).

As a product of Psychoanalysis, the focus of psychodynamic treatment models are the emotional conflicts which are caused by the traumatic experience, not focusing on symptoms alone, but on their meaning. The so-called psychodynamic models of change assert that therapist interventions should promote the expression of avoided affect, the reexperiencing of affect within therapeutic relationship, and the replacement of inappropriate attitudes, expectations and behaviors with more adaptive ones (Town et al., 2017a).

DP has traditionally placed emphasis on insight into relationship patterns and processing avoided emotions, including unconscious thoughts and feelings associated with traumatic events. This technique aims at helping patients to enhance self-understanding, gaining insight into their lives and present-day problems, which may allow them not only to maintain therapeutic improvements but to continue to improve after the end of treatment (Becker et al., 2019). Despite therapist invites the patient to associate freely, he can use interventions to decrease anxiety. "The therapist redirects the patient away from his obsessive thoughts in order to contain affect and prevent him from feeling overwhelmed" (Cabaniss et al., 2011, p. 205). DP works in the connection between reality and unconscious fantasies, through a "free association," or a "free interview," and interpretations of transferential reactions and propensities. It is within the transferential relationship, through the transference-countertransference dynamics, that patient may relive events, thoughts, and feelings, analyzing them and making it possible to elaborate the avoided affects. Furthermore, DP is not only confined to the use of interpretation, but also includes clarification and confrontation as additional therapeutic verbal interventions (Abbass, 2016; Abbass, Kisely, Rasic, and Katzman, 2013; Becker et al., 2019; Hickey, 2015a).

In the 70's and 80's, proposals of DP models appeared, having intersubjectivity as the main focus, such as the Luborsky's supportive-expressive therapy and Davanloo's short-term intensive psychotherapy (ISTDP) (Johansson, Town, and Abbas, 2014; Leichsenting and Steinert, 2017b). The ISTDP, which is a short-term treatment performed in less than 40 sessions, has been shown to be suitable for the treatment of chronic health conditions and fragile character structure, as well as mixed psychiatric disorders (Kenny, Arthey, and Abbass, 2014; Leichsenring and Steinert, 2017; Lilliengren et al., 2017). In general, the first session is longer, consisting of an experimental therapy, or trial therapy, in which a psychodiagnostic evaluation can be performed (Johansson et al., 2014; Town, Abbass, Stride, and Bernier, 2017; Wolff, 2013). In this technique, the path to establishing therapeutic alliance is through overcoming resistances, and the main therapeutic interventions, which aim to unlock the unconscious, include confrontation, clarification, challenge to resistance, head on collision, facilitation of emotional experiences and recapitulation (Becker et al., 2019; Johansson et al., 2014; Wolff, 2013; Abbass, 2016; Abbas et al., 2013; Abbass, Town, Ogrodniczuc, Joffres, and Lilliengren, 2017; Hickey, 2015a; 2015b). The basis of ISTDP is resistance, transference and unconscious therapeutic alliance (Johansson et al., 2014; Hickey, 2015a, 2015b; Hersoug, Hoglend, Gabbard, and Lorentzen, 2012; Hickey, 2015c; 2015d), allowing this technique to be considered an effective treatment, which has been corroborate by studies that cover follow-up interviews and post-treatment assessment measures (Abbas et al., 2017; Ajilchi et al., 2016; Perry, Bond, and Presniak, 2013).

Situations where short-term treatments are required have been the main reason for increasing interest in time-limited psychotherapies, despite doubts that it is possible to do therapy that is both brief and deep. According to Levenson (1995, p. 6), the development of the time-limited dynamic psychotherapy (TLDP) may have been motivated by the fact that, although therapists intend to do a long-term psychotherapy, many of them are driven to do brief therapy, since "most patients choose to stay in therapy only a short time." TLDP, which has its origins in psychodynamic theory and object relations, is an interpersonal brief psychotherapy aimed to provide a new experience and a new understanding for the patients, helping them to modify their relationship patterns, in a maximum of 20 weekly sessions (Levenson, 1995; 2010). Despite this premise, Levenson (1995, p. 45) warned that "the degree to which a patient can comprehend, generalize, and expand on any new understanding is limited by such factors as his or her intellectual ability, capacity for introspection, and psychological-mindedness." Thus, "the therapist needs to take into account the patient´s baseline level of responding and the context of the therapy situation" (p. 205).

Based on a short-term interpersonal model, TLDP may neglect many areas which longer-term therapies address more thoroughly, providing symptomatic relief and leading to personality transformation. While long-term therapists seek change in basic character, following the process of change in the therapeutic setting, TLDP therapists seek to provide patients a new understanding of their interactional style so that they may try out new behaviors in the therapy and then extend to their outside world, considering that therapy continues in the real world (Corey, 2009). TDLP focuses on the most frequently problematic type of interaction of patients, working on it to provide a new experience and understanding, which "is pragmatically essential when time is of the essence" (Levenson, 1995, p. 40). Nevertheless, time seems to be controversial argument, since studies have shown that long-term therapies lead to long-term results, with patients maintaining their state of improvement after the end of therapy (Becker et al., 2019), and TLDP therapists assume that patients may need for additional therapy in the future. As stated by Corey (2009, p. 86), "instead of thinking of TDLP as a definitive intervention, it is best to view this approach as offering multiple, brief therapy experiences over an individual's life span."

In addition to the abovementioned, studies have concluded that "medication had a positive effect on patients' likelihood and capacity to benefit from their short-term therapies" (Levenson, 1995, p. 211), with the combination of TLDP and medication prescription being common. This may raise some doubts about the effectiveness of TLDP, since the improvement observed in patients can be a consequence of the medication effects, and mainly due to "the absence of theoretical and empirical studies examining what happens when a brief psychotherapy ends and the medication monitoring continues" (Levenson, 1995, p. 211).

Studying the effects of psychotherapies has been shown to be a critical issue, especially in the validation of long-term therapies. It is known that short-term DP (here we are not referring to TLDP) have been the subject of empirical studies, presenting outcomes similar to other therapeutic approaches, and even superior in studies that cover follow-up interviews and post-treatment assessment measures (Becker et al., 2019). The outcomes of both the brief and long-term DP are not indistinguishable, but they seek different ends, and long-term treatments are not easily measured, being research on this technique complex and time-consuming (Levenson, 1995).

It is worth mentioning that the first meta-analysis on Long-Term Psychodynamic Psychotherapy (LTPP) was published just over a decade ago by Leichsenring and Rabung (2008), who based their results on RCTs and observational studies published between 1960 and 2008. In order to examine the effects of LTPP, the authors analyzed twenty-three studies involving a total of 1053 patients who had been treated for at least a year, or 50 sessions. Their findings indicated that this technique is an effective treatment for complex disorders, which encompass more than one mental disorder. An update of this meta-analysis was conducted by the same authors (Leichsenring and Rabung, 2011), corroborating the results of the 2008 meta-analysis. In 2014, a review article on empirical evidence of the effectiveness of DP (Leichsenring et al., 2014) was published, presenting results consistent with these previous meta-analyzes. "There is evidence for the efficacy of DP in depressive disorders, prolonged or complicated grief, anxiety disorders, posttraumatic stress disorder, eating disorders, somatic symptom disorders, substance related disorders, and personality disorders" (Leichsenring et al., 2014, p. 119). Briefly, dynamic psychotherapies operate "on an interpretive-supportive continuum. An emphasis is placed on more interpretive or supportive interventions depending on the patient's needs" ((Leichsenring and Rabung, 2008, p. 1552). Therefore, the procedures and components of DP treatment differ according to the specificities of the patient, which precludes the detailed description of the therapeutic process (Landolt and Kenardy, 2015).

## THE TIME IN THE THERAPEUTIC PROCESS

The first treatments conducted by Freud, when investigating hysterical phenomena, were brief and symptom-focused, and he had an active stance with his patients. However, when free association and dream analysis replaced hypnoses method, the treatments became longer (Groves, 1996). The so-called "talking cure" revolutionized the interaction between patient and therapist. The fundamental rule of this method, which is based on free association, is to invite patient to say whatever comes to mind, without restrictions, taking him back to repressed childhood experiences, wishes and fantasies that had resulted in unconscious conflicts.

> The unconscious roots of hitherto irresolvable conflicts that shape the transference-occurrences. [...] With the help of the analyst's interventions – often transference-interpretations of what transpires in the here and now of the session – a new understanding of the patient's suffering will arise. [...] Resolving these conflicts and putting them into perspective or at rest will free the patient's mind from old inhibitions and make room for new choices. (IPA, "About Psychoanalysis")

The exploration of the transference replaced direct suggestion, and the interaction of the therapist with the patient substantially decreased, reasons for which the analysis growing longer and longer (Groves, 1996). As before mentioned, the first movements to shorten the therapeutic process of psychoanalysis, after recognizing the role of the transferential relationship, date back to the beginning of its formal practice, with the active technique proposed by Ferenczi. Since then, the history of psychoanalysis has been circulating between short-term and long-term therapies.

Although Freud is known as an apologist of time as the possibility of accessing the deeper layers of psychic development, which can lead to finding solutions to current problems, reducing the time for subsequent treatments in the case of an equally serious illness and thus, gradually overcoming the timelessness of the unconscious, it is worth mentioning that there were occasions when he chose to limit the duration of treatments. It does not mean that Freud was adopting short-term therapy, since he was shortening the time of the analytical processes when identifying feasibility issues. "In this setting, the time restrictions are purely set out of pragmatic reasons external to the therapeutic process and have little to do with altering or ameliorating this process" (De Geest and Megank, 2019, p. 208).

Brief therapies, which have a predetermined duration, are symptom-focused and rely on an active stance of the therapist, are controversial. According to a recent theoretical review (De Geest and Megank, 2019), several authors have agreed that the application of a time limit is one of the features that enables an acceleration of therapeutic change, as it is believed that therapists and patients are encouraged to work harder and faster with the deadline in sight. On the other hand, the pressure of time can lead to the choice of an inappropriate focus, and work can be conducted superficially, without addressing crucial issues. Although De Geest and Megank (2019, p. 217) have not come to a definitive conclusion, as studies have suggested that "a time limit sets pressure on the therapy process and creates a kind of expectancy effect, which can have both negative and positive consequences," their findings indicated that should be taken into account that there is no type of therapy suitable for all patients, with time being a relevant factor that interacts with the variations in the therapeutic processes.

As previously mentioned, the therapy must be conducted considering the treatment's goals and, mainly, the patient's capacity to process and tolerate feelings, which reflects directly on the length of therapy. The nuances of the time in the therapeutic process are now discussed through clinical vignettes. The following vignettes describe cases in which a time limit has not been set and, although they are longer than other psychotherapies, the cases can be considered short-term therapies, as they do not exceed 40 sessions (Becker et al., 2019; Lilliengren et al., 2017).

## Vignette 1

When Anna arrived for the first session of therapy she was a 32-year-old single woman. In the first session, in which a psychodiagnostic evaluation was performed, Anna said that she was raped more than a decade ago, without clearly explaining what happened. She only said that this experience took her to isolation for 3 years. In this period of isolation, Anna became involved with a person she met online, which led to another experience described as complicated. She said she went to another city to meet this person and the situation she experienced made her realize that it could be a sex trafficking network. Anna's speech was confusing, she vaguely described these experiences,. Through this session, Anna mentioned having sleep problems, that she related to work, said that she suffered from severe back pain, emphasizing not having "excellent health." It was the worsening of her back pain that led her to resign at the previous work. At the time she began the therapy, Anna was unemployed, working in an institution due to a professional insertion program promoted by the government.

The beginning of the treatment essentially involved anxiety regulation and the establishment of a good therapeutic alliance. The aim of the therapy was to increase insight about Anna's subjective experiences of relational distress, identifying her defensive system and its consequences in her life. The therapeutic process served to interpret the communication of patient's symptoms, exploring the associated feelings to contain them. Although Anna did not miss the therapy sessions, she did not address or even avoided subjects that might appear related to the rape. On the other hand, other adversities faced in childhood and adolescence were gradually reported in the first months of treatment. Bullying at school and a poor health were described as a summary of her growing. Regarding her health, Anna mentioned that since she was a child she suffered from allergies, stomach pains, headaches, fatigue, and dizziness, needing to visit health centers, take medication and undergo clinical examinations. Health concerns were recurrent theme of Anna's sessions who mentioned lack of attention and perception of the body signs, neglect of symptoms, poor diet and behaviors that aggravated symptoms.

Throughout therapy, the therapist encouraged Anna to explore psychosocial stressors and the possible role of emotional factors in contributing to the development and maintenance of her symptoms. Experiencing and processing unresolved feelings was central in the Anna's therapy. Emotional awareness and augmenting self-reflection capacity and anxiety tolerance allowed the patient to integrate the emotional state which was predisposing and perpetuating her vulnerability to somatic distress. In the seventh month of therapy, Anna was able to talk about bullying she had suffered at school and the death of relatives, whom she cared for in the last months of their lives, without crying. The patient said she was impressed, and that it was the "attempt to stop forgetting" that was allowing her to deal with her griefs.

In the ninth month of treatment, differently of the beginning of the treatment, Anna began related the stressful situations and her emotional state to the symptoms or, at least, to her health perception, saying that sometimes she realized that "focusing on symptoms was a way of not thinking about other issues." In this period, Anna began to talk about her difficulty in maintaining a relationship, her feeling of "suffocation" with the presence of the last boyfriend, with whom it was not clear whether she had sexual involvement. The therapist perceived in Anna's speech a permission, perhaps even a request, to address the rape event. It was as if the patient said she was ready to face her unresolved experiences and feelings. Anna described the rape, her feelings about the fact and its consequences, including online involvement with a person who deceived her. In the session following the description of the rape, Anna arrived at the therapy with an expression that seemed she was relieved, she was calm and smiling, and told a dream she had after that session: "I was a

> child and riding a bicycle on the street with a boy. We were both smiling, and it looked like he was my boyfriend. So, I took my feet off the bike. I felt free and happy in that dream." The therapist and Anna reflected on what the dream represented, and Anna said that the most difficult subject was addressed at the proper time. Anna emphasized that the whole therapeutic process was necessary so that she could see the adversities she faced in a different way; in a way she could deal with. At the end of 1 year of weekly sessions, Anna was able to talk about sexuality, including her expectations about relationships, her symptoms significantly decrease, and she had established and achieved professional goals. The treatment lasted 12 months, and the three-month follow-up interview indicated that Anna continued to improve after the end of the therapy.

Anna's treatment was based on experiencing and processing her unresolved feelings, identifying her behavioral and thought patterns, as well as the anxiety triggers. The interventions were used to detect, clarify, and challenge avoidance strategies that led Anna to somatic distress. Through interpretative interventions, the therapist allowed Anna to make the link between symptoms and emotional state, encouraging her to deal with traumatic memories and hidden emotions. Furthermore, time was a crucial factor of Anna's treatment. Although the therapist did not set a time limit for her treatment, attempts were made to explore the feelings aroused by the patient's traumatic experiences in order to identify the triggers for her symptoms. The patient made it clear that she needed time, time to remember and even more time to be able to repeat and elaborate those experiences.

In the beginning of her treatment, Anna was unable to talk about thoughts and feelings, as often observed in patients with somatic symptoms, she described facts and symptoms. Her desires were put aside for a long time and, considering that, we can say that it did not take long for her to start becoming aware of them. It took her time. Disclosing to the patient the symptom as a resistance to therapy and, more than that, as her means of avoiding dealing with the adversities that arose throughout her life, allowed the progress of the treatment. As stated by Freud (1914), giving the patient time to face the resistance, elaborating it, overcoming it, and continuing the therapeutic process despite it, is a fundamental rule of the therapy.

Through the treatment of his patients, Freud realized that the mind was an ever-changing system, and most of its activities took place outside consciousness. "Unconscious mental activity affects conscious thoughts, feelings, and behaviors" (Cabaniss et al., 2011, p. 4). Psychoanalytic treatment aims to access these unconscious elements to find a solution to patients' symptoms. However, "it must to be careful not give a patient the solution of a symptom or the translation of a wish until he is already so close to it that he has only one short step more to make in order to get hold of the explanation for himself" (Freud, 1912, p. 140). This statement considers that the knowledge of the unconscious content is not enough to eliminate symptoms, it is imperative to overcome resistance. Resistance is anything that opposes the work of the treatment. "Anything can function as resistance – silence, hiding feelings, being too agreeable, missing sessions, not paying one's bills – anything" (Cabaniss et al., 2011, p. 205). As stated by Freud (1914, p. 155), "this working-through of the resistances may in practice turn out to be an arduous task for the subject of the analysis and a trial of patience for the analyst. Nevertheless it is a part of the work which effects the greatest changes in the patient."

## Vignette 2

> Lucas was a 35-years old volunteer firefighter who decided to see a therapist due to have a set of symptoms of post-traumatic stress such as nightmares, intrusive thoughts, irritability, startle reactions, and avoidance behaviors, which were causing significant impairment in his affective and professional life. Although he started his therapy by talking about the violent forest fires he had faced in the previous year, which was one of the subjects of his nightmares, a road accident that occurred five years earlier had emerged as the trigger for the first symptoms of post-traumatic stress. Lucas described his reaction when he arrived at the accident scene by saying he "froze" when he saw the bus under the ravine and only came to his sense when a colleague pushed him to start to help

the victims. This event took him away from the fire department, as being on duty caused him great distress. At that moment, Lucas sought a psychologist who advised him to gradually return to spend time with his fellow firefighters and, in a few months, Lucas resumed his activities. However, the nightmares continued and "down moments" became part of his life. In that time, Lucas never went into therapy; he said he only saw the psychologist twice and exchanged text messages.

In the first sessions of his therapy, Lucas presented detailed reports on the road accidents and the forest fires from the previous year. As the summer approached, the focus of his therapy became the fear of fires, but also his interpersonal relationships, with conflicts being due to Lucas's irritability and aggressivity. More than the current traumatic experiences, therapy was focused on patient's interpretation of the conflicts he had with family members and co-workers and the feelings when he was under stress, which brought back memories of his childhood, family relationships and the unsatisfied need to meet his father's expectations. Lucas reported that his father doubted that he could become a firefighter, as he was afraid of fire as a child and he was an unmotivated teenager, who spent time at the bar drinking with friends. He said his father did not appreciate him, despite being the only son who gained financial independence and needed no help from him. Patient's relationship with his father seemed to be behind his conflicts. The feeling of impotence when he froze in the ravine revealed to be the trigger of his symptoms, heightened by anguish when facing the violent forest fires, which led Lucas to relive the fear of fire felt in childhood and, thus, the consequent feeling of disappointing his father.

In the first months, Lucas's reports were focused on the road accident and the violence of the fires, in an attempt to show how he faced dangerous and interesting situations. Paying attention to countertransference proved to be crucial for the therapist, who perceived a dramatic tone in the patient's speech, as if he were describing an action movie, where the greatest pleasure was in reporting the most tense scenes. The therapist's stance allowed Lucas to leave his "ideal speech" and face his feelings of helplessness and incompetence with which he had been struggling since childhood. As the therapy progressed, and Lucas tried to deal with his memories and feelings, there was a moment of withdrawal. Lucas went back to talking about conflicts in the firefighters' routine, this time emphasizing the role of women in disrupting the work environment. As the therapist was a woman, Lucas quickly explained that he had nothing against women and emphasized that he hoped the therapist had not misunderstood him. Lucas said the male firefighters have also changed and the blame for the problem in the fire department was also on the men. In the same session, he reported on his girlfriend's behavior and how much she upset him, demanding arrangements at their home. At that moment, the therapist said: "apparently women change your entire environment." Lucas smiled and agreed saying that his girlfriend "wanted to change everything" and, if it was like that in the beginning, he believed she could drive him crazy." The choice of words and the feeling conveyed meant the therapist did not intervene directly, which could be done. In the next session, the patient resumed the path of therapy and, perhaps, feeling that he was able to do this without explicit help was important for his therapeutic process.

A crucial moment in Lucas's therapeutic process was when he associated the anger he felt towards a colleague who was unable to act properly when fighting a forest fire with his performance in the road accident (when he froze in the ravine), linking the feelings aroused to the relationship with his father. Through therapy, the therapist encouraged Lucas to face the feelings of helplessness and the anger he transferred to people around him. The need to set his own goals and realize that the expectations he believed his father, girlfriend, or even the therapist had about him could be a way to reduce the anxiety produced by his feelings of guilt and failure. Emotional awareness and an increased capacity for self-reflection allowed Lucas to integrate the emotional state, to identify stress triggers and to elaborate feelings regarding their childhood experiences. In the eighth month of treatment, Lucas no longer presented symptoms of post-traumatic stress, even in the face of new adversities such as paternity, changes in the functioning of the fire department, firefighting, and rescue of critical victims. The treatment lasted 9 months, and the three-month follow-up interview indicated that Lucas maintained his state of improvement, without presenting post-traumatic stress symptoms and with a better quality of life.

Lucas's therapy was initially based on addressing maladaptive defense mechanisms that could be arousing his symptoms, helping him to unveil the meaning of the traumatic events. The road accident and forest fires led Lucas to relive his childhood experiences, with feelings of helplessness and guilt being the main reasons for the patient's psychic disorganization. The treatment of traumatic stress symptoms, through DP:

> [...] seeks to foster insights about factors that create hypersensitivity to overt and covert trauma reminders. Thus, the goals of psychodynamic trauma therapy include bringing unconscious material into awareness; establishing a sense of meaning, purpose, and safety; examining affects such as guilt and shame; fostering insights into how threatening thoughts and feelings are kept from awareness in order to reduce hyperarousal; and examining the therapeutic relationship for symbolic reenactments of past trauma. (D'Andrea and Pole, 2012, p. 438)

The transferential relationship was an important aspect of Lucas's therapy, as he seemed committed to meeting the expectations he thought the therapist had, with a demand to be recognized for his bravery in the face of his dangerous duties. In addition, when talking about the problems that women caused in his life, transference feelings were presented as stories about significant others, as a way of telling therapist that she was disturbing his mind. In both situations, the therapist chose to approach the transference feelings within the context brought by the patient, recognizing that Lucas needed time to overcome such resistance. "It often makes sense to explore them [transference feelings] in the displacement before confronting the transference. This allows therapist to learn more about the feelings while the patient is talking about them in a more comfortable sphere" (Cabaniss et al., 2011, p. 224).

Lucas presented a weakened ego function, requiring the therapist, at the beginning of the treatment, to use supporting interventions. As highlighted by Cabaniss et al. (2011, p. 228), "showing the patient that you can tolerate their strong feelings without judging them, becoming upset, or causing a rupture in the treatment is one of the most critical features of the 'holding function' of psychotherapy." Thus, initially the focus of Lucas's therapy was on the therapeutic alliance, crucial to his adherence to treatment. Subsequently, the uncovering interventions became part of his therapeutic process, with confrontation and clarification being the most effective ones.

Time, especially for the construction and improvement of the therapeutic alliance, was essential for the success of Lucas's treatment. The active stance of the therapist, without disrespecting the patient's subjectivity, allowed Lucas to achieve emotional awareness and an increased capacity of self-reflection, helping him to identify stress triggers and develop internal resources to deal with possible future stressful events. The emotional awareness, reconstruction of warded-off memories, and meaning-making "may have slowed down automatic processing of trauma stimuli and enhance emotion regulation in the face of such cues" (D'Andrea and Pole, 2012, p. 444).

## Conclusion

Psychotherapies based on psychoanalytic theory have been studied for more than a century, with attempts to shorten therapeutic processes without impairing the focus on unconscious processes and the meaning of symptoms. Time has proved to be an important factor, especially because it is considered an obstacle to scientific research aimed at validating the effectiveness of psychotherapies, which seems to be the main reason why DP remains outside the front-line of treatments for mental disorders. However, more than finding express solutions to their symptoms and conflicts, patients are interested in long-term results, which DP seems to achieve. Through the processing of avoided emotions, the reexperiencing of affects within therapeutic relationship, and the replacement of inappropriate attitudes, expectations and behaviors with more adaptative ones, this technique seeks symptomatic relief, while helping patients to enhance self-understanding, gaining insight into their lives and present-day problems, which may allow them to maintain therapeutic improvements, or even to continue to improve after the end of treatment.

Time, often considered an enemy, in this chapter proves to be an ally of the therapeutic process. In the cases presented through clinical vignettes, time was an essential tool for the success of treatments: time for the establishment of the therapeutic alliance, time for the working-through resistance, time to face traumatic memories, which led to the resolution of inner conflicts and overcoming of symptoms. Therapy must be tailored to the patient's capacity to process and tolerate feelings, to elaborate and overcome the resistance, stages that are part of the process that leads him/her to achieve the treatment goals. It is worth emphasizing that time is a continuous process of the patient's growth, which does not stop with the end of therapy.

## References


Abbass, A. (2016). The Emergence of Psychodynamic Psychotherapy for Treatment Resistant Patients: Intensive Short-Term Dynamic Psychotherapy. *Psychodynamic Psychiatry*, 44(2): 245–280. doi: 10.1521/pdps.2016.44.2.245.

Abbass, A., Kisely, S., Rasic, D., and Katzman, J. W. (2013). Residency Training in Intensive Short-Term Dynamic Psychotherapy: Methods and Cost-Effectiveness. *Psychiatric Annals*, 43(11): 508-512. doi: 10.3928/00485713-20131105-06.

Abbas, A., Town, J., Ogrodniczuk, J., Joffres, M., and Lilliengren, P. (2017). Intensive Short-Term Dynamic Psychotherapy Trial Therapy: Effectiveness and Role of "Unlocking the Unconscious." *J Nerv Ment Dis*, 205 (6): 453-457. doi: 10.1097/NMD.0000000000000684.

Ajilchi, B., Nejati, V., Town, J., Wilson, R., and Abbass, A. (2016). Effects of Intensive Short-Term Dynamic Psychotherapy on Depressive Symptoms and Executive Functioning in Major Depression. *J Nerv Ment Dis,* 204: 500-505. doi: 10.1097/NMD.0000000000000518.

Aragão Oliveira, R., and Oliveira, S. S. (2012). Sobre a investigação do processo terapêutico em Psicanálise e em Psicoterapia Dinâmica. *Revista Portuguesa de Psicanálise*, 32 (2): 43-57. [The investigation of the therapeutic process in Psychoanalysis and Psychoanalytic Psychotherapy. *Portuguese Psychoanalytic Journal,* 32 (2): 43-57].

Batista, L. C., Senra, H., and Aragão Oliveira, R. (2014). A relação terapêutica na psicoterapia psicanalítica: experiências vividas por ex-pacientes. *R B Psicoterapia,* 16 (3): 1-15. [The therapeutic relationship in psychoanalytic psychotherapy: experiences of former patients. *R B Psicoterapia,* 16 (3): 1-15].

Becker, J. P., Paixão, R., Silva, Simone S., Quartilho, M. J., and Custódio, E. M. (2019). Dynamic Psychotherapy: The Therapeutic Process in the Treatment of Obsessive-Compulsive Disorder. *Behavioral Sciences*, 9 (12): 141. doi: 10.3390/bs9120141.

Breuer, J. and Freud, S. (1893). Studies on Hysteria. In *The Standard Edition of the Complete Psychological Works of Sigmund Freud Vol II (1893-1895): Studies on Hysteria.* London: The Hogarth Press and the Institute of Psycho-Analysis, 1955.

Cabaniss, D., Cherry, S., Douglas, C., and Schwartz, A. (2011). *Psychodynamic Psychotherapy: A Clinical Manual.* New York: Wiley-Blackwell.

Chavooshi, B., Saberi, M., Tavallaie, S. A., and Sahraei, H. (2017). Psychotherapy for Medically Unexplained Pain: A Randomized Clinical Trial Comparing Intensive Short-Term Dynamic Psychotherapy and Cognitive Behavior Therapy. *Psychosomatics,* 58 (5): 506-518. doi: 10.1016/j.psym.2017.01.003.

Conci, M. (2019). Ferenczi and Freud – From psychoanalysis as a "professional and personal home" to the creation of a "psychoanalytic home" for the patient. *International Forum of Psychoanalysis*, 28 (4): 193-202. doi: 10.1080/0803706X. 2019.1643038.

Corey, G. (2009). *Theory and Practice of Counseling and Psychotherapy.* Belmont, CA: Thomson Brooks/Cole.

D'Andrea, W., and Pole, N. (2012). A Naturalistic Study of the Relation Of Psychotherapy Process to Change in Symptoms, Information Processing, and Physiological Activity in Complex Trauma. *Psychol Trauma,* 4 (4), 438-446. doi: 10.1037/a0025067.

De Geest, R. M., and Meganck, R. (2019). How Do Time Limits Affect Our Psychotherapies? A Literature Reviwe. *Psychologica Belgica*, 59 (1): 206-226. doi: 10.5334/pb.475.

Evans, S. C., Roberts, M. C., Keeley, J. W., Blossom, J. B., Amaro, C. M., Garcia, A. M., Stough, C. O., Canter, K. S., Robles, R., and Reed, G. M. (2015). Vignette methodologies for studying clinicians' decision-making: Validity, utility, and application in ICD-11 field studies. *Int J Clin Health Psychol,* 15(2): 160-170. doi: 10.1016/ j.ijchp.2014.12.001 .

Ferenczi, S., and Rank, O. (1925). *The development of psychoanalysis.* Madison, CT: International Universities Press, 1986.

Fonagy, P. (2015). The effectiveness of psychodynamic psychotherapies: na update. *World Psychiatry,* 14: 137-150. doi: 10.1002/wps.20235.

Freud, S. (1913a). Princípios Básicos da Psicanálise. In *Sigmund Freud Obras Completas Vol 10: Observações psicanalíticas sobre um caso de paranoia relatado em autobiografia ("O caso Schreber"), Artigos sobre a Técnica e outros textos,* 204-211. São Paulo: Companhia das Letras, 2010. [On Psycho-Analysis. In *The Complete Works of Sigmund Freud, The Vol 10: psychoanalytical observations* on a case of paranoia reported through autobiography *("The Case of Schreber"), Paper on Technique and Other Works.* 204-211. São Paulo: Companhia das Letras, 2010].

Freud, S. (1913b). On Beginning the Treatment. In *The Standard Edition of the Complete Psychological Works of Sigmund Freud Vol XII (1911-1913): The Case of Schreber, Papers on Technique and Other Works.* 123-144. London: The Hogarth Press and the Institute of Psycho-Analysis, 1958.

Freud (1936 [1926]) Inhibitions, Symptoms and Anxiety. *The Psychoanalytic Quarterly*, 5(1): 1-28. doi: 10.1080/21674086. 1936.11925270.

Freud, S. (1921). Psicologia das Massas e Análise do Eu. In *Sigmund Freud Obras Completas Vol 15: Psicologia das Massas e Análise do Eu e Outros Textos*, 9-100. São Paulo: Companhia das Letras, 2011. [Group Psychology and the Analysis of the Ego. In *The Complete Works of Sigmund Freud, The Vol 15: Group Psychology and Analysis of the Ego and Other Works,* 9-100. São Paulo: Companhia das Letras, 2011].

Freud, S. (1912). Recomendações ao Médico que Pratica a Psicanálise. In *Sigmund Freud Obras Completas Vol 10: Observações psicanalíticas sobre um caso de paranoia relatado em autobiografia ("O caso Schreber"), Artigos sobre a Técnica e outros textos,* 111-122. São Paulo: Companhia das Letras, 2010. [Recomendations to Physicians Practising Psycho-Analysis. In *The Complete Works of Sigmund Freud, The Vol 10: psychoanalytical observations* on a case of paranoia reported through autobiography *("The Case of Schreber"), Paper on Technique and Other Works,* 111-122. São Paulo: Companhia das Letras, 2010].

Freud, S. (1918). História de uma neurose infantil ("O Homem dos Lobos," 1918 [1914]). In *Sigmund Freud Obras Completas Vol 14: História de uma neurose infantil ("O Homem dos Lobos"), Além do Princípio do Prazer e outros textos,* 9-119. São Paulo: Companhia das Letras, 2010. [From the History of na Infantile Neurosis ("The Wolf Man," 1918[1914]. In *The Complete Works of Sigmund Freud, The Vol 14: From the History of na Infantile Neurosis ("The Wolf Man"), Beyond* the *Pleasure Principle and Other Works, 9-119.* São Paulo: Companhia das Letras, 2010].

Freud, S. (1914). Remembering, Repeating and Working-Through. In *The Standard Edition of the Complete Psychological Works of Sigmund Freud Vol XII (1911-1913): The Case of Schreber, Papers on Technique and Other Works.* 147-156. London: The Hogarth Press and the Institute of Psycho-Analysis, 1958.

Gabbard, G. O. (2014). Treatment in Dynamic Psychiatry - Individual Psychotherapy. In *Psychodynamic Psychiatry in Clinical Practice*, edited by Glen O. Gabbard, 94-134. Washington, DC: American Psychiatric Press.

Groves, J. E. (1996). Introduction: Four "Essences" of Short-Term Therapy: Brevity, Focus, Activity, Selectivity. In *Essential Papers on Short-Term Dynamic Therapy*, edited by James E. Groves, 1-25. New York: New York University Press.

Hersoug, A. G., Hoglend, P., Gabbard, G. O., and Lorentzen, S. (2012). The combined predictive effect of patient characteristics and alliance on long-term dynamic and interpersonal functioning after dynamic psychotherapy. *Clin Psychol Psychother*, 20 (4): 297-307. doi: 10.1002/cpp.1770.

Hickey, C. M. (2015a). Multidimensional unconscious structural changes in Davanloo's intensive short-term dynamic psychotherapy. Part I. *Archives of Psychiatry and Psychotherapy*, 1: 45–51. doi: 10.12740/APP/36560.

Hickey, C. M. (2015b). Multidimensional unconscious structural changes in Davanloo's intensive short-term dynamic psychotherapy. Part II. *Archives of Psychiatry and Psychotherapy*, 1: 53–57. doi: 10.12740/APP/36563.

Hickey, C. M. (2015c). The Major Mobilization of the Unconscious and the Total Removal of Resistance in Davanloo's Intensive Short-term Dynamic Psychotherapy. Part I: An Introduction. *Am J Psychother,* 69 (4): 423-439. doi: 10.1176/appi.psychotherapy.2015.69.4.423.

Hickey, C. M. (2015d). The Major Mobilization of the Unconscious and the Total Removal of Resistance in Davanloo's Intensive Short-term Dynamic Psychotherapy Part II: Treating the Transference Neurosis. *Am J Psychother*, 69 (4): 441-454. doi: 10.1176/appi.psychotherapy.2015.69.4.441.

International Psychoanalytical Association (IPA). About Psychoanalysis. Accessed August 17, 2020. https://www.ipa.world/ipa/en/Psychoanalysis/en/Psychoanalysis/Psychoanalysis.aspx.

Johansson, R., Town, J. M., and Abbass, A. (2014). Davanloo's Intensive Short-Term Dynamic Psychotherapy in a tertiary psychotherapy service: overall effectiveness and association between unlocking the unconscious and outcome. *Peer J*, 2: e548. doi: 10.7717/peerj.548.

Kenny, D. T., Arthey, S., and Abbass, A. (2014). Intensive Short-Term Dynamic Psychotherapy for Severe Music Performance Anxiety. *Med Probl Perform Art*, 29 (1): 3-7. doi:10.21091/mppa.2014.1002.

Landolt, M., and Kenardy, J. (2015). Evidence-Based Treatments for Children and Adolescents. In *Evidence Based Treatments for Trauma-Related Psychological Disorders: A Practical Guide for Clinicians*, edited by Ulrich Schnyder and Marylène Cloitre, 363-380). Zurich: Springer.

Leichsenring, F. (2005). Are psychodynamic and psychoanalytic therapies effective? A review of empirical data. *The International Journal of Psychoanalysis,* 86 (3): 841-868. doi: 10.1516/RFEE-LKPN-B7TF-KPDU.

Leichsenring, F., Klein, S., and Salzer, S. (2014). The Efficacy of Psychodynamic Psychotherapy in Specific Mental Disorders: A 2013 Update of Empirical Evidence. *Contemporary Psychoanalysis,* 50 (1-2): 89-130. doi: 10.1080/00107530.2014.880310.

Leichsenring, F., and Rabung, S. (2008). Effectiveness of Long-Term Psychodynamic Psychotherapy: A Meta-analysis. *JAMA,* 300 (13): 1551-1565. doi: 10.1001/jama.300.13.1551.

Leichsenring, F., and Rabung, S. (2011). Long-term psychodynamic psychotherapyin complex mental disorders: Update of a meta-analysis. *British Journal of Psychiatry*, 199 (1): 15–22. doi: 10.1192/bjp.bp.110.082776 .

Leichsenring F., and Steinert, C. (2017). Short-term psychodynamic therapy for obsessive-compulsive disorder: A manual-guided approach to treating the "inhibited rebel." *Bull Menninger Clin*, 81 (4): 1–49. doi: 10.1521/bumc_2017_81_07.

Levenson, H. (2010). *Brief Dynamic Therapy*. Washington, DC: American Psychological Association.

Levenson, H. (1995). *Time-Limited Dynamic Psychotherapy: A Guide to Clinical Practice*. New York: Basic Books.

Levi, O., Bar-Haim, Y., Kreiss, Y., and Fruchter, E. (2015). Cognitive-Behavioural Therapy and Psychodynamic Psychotherapy in the Treatment of Combat-Related Post-Traumatic Stress Disorder: A Comparative Efecctiveness Study. *Clin Psychol Psychother,* 23 (4): 298-307. doi: 10.1002/cpp.1969.

Lilliengren, P., Johansson, R., Town, J., Kisely, S., and Abbass, A. (2017). Intensive Short-Term Dynamic Psychotherapy for generalized anxiety disorder: A pilot effectiveness and process-outcome study. *Clin Psychol Psychother,* 24 (6): 1313-1321. doi: 10.1002/cpp.2101.

Ness, E., Dahl, H. J., Talberg, P., Amlo, S., Høglend, P., Thorén, A., Egeland, J., and Ulberg, R. (2018). Assessment of dynamic change in psychotherapy with adolescentes. *Child Adolesc Psychiatry Ment Health,* 12 (39). doi: 10.1186/s13034-018-0246-z.

Paixão, R. (2006). Inventário das Expectativas sobre a Psicoterapia: primeiros estudos da versão portuguesa do "Psychotherapy Expectancy Inventory-R." *Psychologica*, 43: 175-192. [Psychotherapy Expectancy Inventory-R - First Study for the Portuguese Population. *Psychologica*, 43: 175-192].

Paixão, R., and Nunes, J. (2008). Adaptação Portuguesa da Escala de Aliança Psicoterapêutica da Califórnia (versão do paciente). *Revista Toxicodependências,* 14 (2): 75-78. [Portuguese Adaptation of the California Psychotherapy Alliance Scale (patient's version). *Revista Toxicodependências,* 14 (2): 75-78].

Perry, J. C., Bond, M., and Presniak, M. D. (2013). Alliance, reactions to treatment, and counter-transference in the process of recovery from suicidal phenomena in long-term dynamic psychotherapy. *Psychotherapy Research*, 23 (5): 592-605. doi: 10.1080/10503307.2013.809560.

Perry, J. C., Bond, M., and Békés, V. (2017). The Rate of Improvement in Long-Term Dynamic Psychotherapy for Borderline Personality Disorder. *J Nerv Ment Dis,* 205 (7): 517-524 doi: 10.1097/NMD.0000000000000697.

Sifneos, P. (1979). *Short-Term Dynamic Psychotherapy: Evaluation and Technique*. New York: Plenum Medical Book Company.

Town, J. M., Salvadori, A., Falkenström, F., Bradley, S., and Hardy, G. (2017a). Is affect experiencing therapeutic in major depressive disorder? Examining associations between affect experiencing and changes to the aliance and outcome in intensive short-term dynamic psychotherapy. *Psychotherapy,* 54 (2): 148-158. doi: 10.1037/ pst0000108 .

Town, J. M., Abbas, A., Stride, C., and Bernier, D. (2017b). A randomised controlled trial of Intensive Short- Term Dynamic Psychotherapy for treatment resistant depression: the Halifax Depression Study. *J Affect Disord*, 214: 15-25. doi: 10.1016/j.jad.2017.02.035.

Wolff, D. M. (2013). Intensive Short-Term Dynamic Psychotherapy in the Private Practice of Psychiatry. *Psychiatric Annals*, 43(11): 491-495. doi: 10.3928/00485713-20131105-03.

In: Psychotherapy
Editor: Hayley Boyd
ISBN: 978-1-53618-877-6


*Chapter 4*

# THE CURATIVE POWER OF HAPPY SCIENCE RELIGIOUS INTERVENTION (PRAYER) ON COVID-19

***Yoichi Chida***[1,2,*]***, MD, PhD***
[1]Faculty of Human Happiness, Happy Science University, Chosei, Chiba, Japan
[2]Department of Medical Science, Happy Smile Clinic, Kawasaki, Kanagawa, Japan

## ABSTRACT

Recent decades have seen a tremendous increase in scientific interest regarding the relationship between religion and health. In particular, and in regard to the impact of the Wuhan Coronavirus Disease (COVID-19), the putative effectiveness of religious intervention on infectious diseases has received greater attention worldwide. Indeed, Hummer et al., (2010) analyzed data from a 16-year prospective study of a US representative sample of 20,139 cases, of whom 3,934 were identified as having died. People who attended religious services more than once a week exhibited

* Corresponding Author's E-mail: yoichi.chida@gmail.com.

less than half the risk of death due to infectious disease in the follow-up period compared with those who had never attended. Our research group has previously reported randomized clinical trials in which a group psychotherapy or prayer based on Happy Science – a religious movement founded by Master Ryuho Okawa in 1986 that has since grown into one of the most influential religious organizations in Japan – doctrine significantly reduces depressive symptoms, which robustly deteriorate a wide range of physical disorders. Moreover, Happy Science has recently published some clinical cases in which Happy Science prayers cured COVID-19. Thus, this article reviews previous reports showing the ameliorating effects of religious interventions on infectious diseases and suggests possible underlying mechanisms.

## 1. Introduction and Happy Science

Historically, there has been a strong connection between religion and medicine (Koenig, 2012). In the West, the church built the first public hospitals in as early as the fourth century; furthermore, it was religious orders that trained and registered doctors, right up until the time of the Reformation. However, beginning in the seventeenth century – and the time of the Enlightenment –a nearly total separation developed between religion and medicine, as evidenced by the widespread global cultural turn towards science and technology for explanations of disease and healing. From this time onward, there has been a major focus on the physical management of disease, which has left spiritual or psychological approaches as secondary considerations – at best, they are deemed as alternatives or complementary forms of medicine. Nonetheless, in more recent times, the perception concerning this separation has benefitted from the returning swing of the pendulum, of sorts.

The Wuhan Coronavirus Disease (COVID-19), since its emergence, has resulted in a large number of deaths worldwide but has not yet seen any efficient vaccines and/or medicines for its treatment. As such, the putative effectiveness of religious intervention has received greater attention from all over the world. Thus, this article reviews previous research on religion and infectious diseases and, more intriguingly, reports that Happy Science prayers cured COVID-19 in some cases. In light of this, we suggest possible underlying mechanisms.

Before moving on to discussing the main tenets of this paper, Happy Science is briefly described and explained. Happy Science – originally established in Japan as "Kofuku-no-Kagaku" (lit., the Science of Human Happiness) in 1986 – has grown into one of the most influential religious organizations in Japan, and now includes a global following with members from over 100 different countries. Master Ryuho Okawa (founder and leader of Happy Science) has, as of July 2020, presented more than 3,100 lectures (including over 150 lectures in English) and published over 2,700 books (in over 31 different languages). His lectures cover a large range of genres and topics, including spirituality, health and medical care, science, human relationships, business and economy, politics, and education (Happy Science, 2020a).

The basic tenets of Happy Science, and the core of its teachings, are known as "The Principles of Happiness," which consist of the fourfold path of "Love," "Wisdom," "Self-reflection," and "Progress" (Okawa, 2009). Based on these principles, Happy Science has developed a novel religious/spiritual group psychotherapy, and has reported its efficacy in relation to various mental disorders via randomized controlled trials (Chida & Kim, 2011; Chida et al., 2016). Happy Science believers receive a sutra book – "The Dharma of the Right Mind" – and a set of prayer books. "The Dharma of the Right Mind" was inspired by Shakyamuni Buddha's consciousness and therefore has the power to purify minds with the light of Buddha. This prayer has been described as possessing 10,000 times more power than the Lotus Sutra or the Heart Sutra of Buddhism (Happy Science, 2020a). Happy Science members' spiritual life, of which prayer constitutes a core component, revolves around the recitation of the sutras and prayers contained in these books.

Happy Science has a unique cosmology. It is believed that the universe has a multi-dimensional structure. Within this structure, the material world is three-dimensional, whereas the other world – the spirit world – refers to the fourth dimension and above. The spirit world of planet Earth continues to the Ninth dimension, which is the highest limit of personified spiritual existence. Followers of Happy Science believe in the existence of the Supreme Being, known as El Cantare, whose existence is similar to that which many religions – such as Christianity and Islam – refer to as God. El Cantare is the leader of ten ninth-dimension spirits, including Jesus Christ, Confucius, Zeus, and Moses (Okawa, 2013). Indeed, Master Ryuho Okawa has offered many teachings on this fact, including the following (Okawa, 2008b):

> "It was I who was guiding Jesus. He referred to me as 'Father,' and prayed to me every day. [...] Some 2,500 years ago, I sent one of my brother souls, Shakyamuni Buddha to earth. I also sent Mohammed, the founder of Islam, to Earth. Then, I created a band of more than 40 angels, who were directed to give Mohammed guidance. [...] However, standing behind this band of angels and directing their communication was, in fact, El Cantare, who appointed Archangel Gabriel to be the communicator, and it is Gabriel (Jibril), who was largely responsible for the transmissions. In short, it was I who provided guidance for Buddhism, Christianity, and Islam – every one of them. I also guided Moses. [...] I can summon any deity, high-level spirit, or angel. [...] However, if I summon any high spirit – whether they are the saints and sages of Christianity, Shinto, or Buddhism – they cannot deny me. I am capable of receiving spiritual messages from all factions of religion. This is the position of El Cantare. In other words, I am their 'Master', and I am in the position of directing them. [...] Consequently, Happy Science must – logically and inevitably – grow larger into a world religion. We have the mission to unite all the world's religions into one. It is, by reason and logic, our duty. [...] I am not using it in the sense of the 'Master of Japanese people'. Rather, it is in reference to my mission to lead all humankind in unity."

In the Happy Science cosmology, human souls repeat reincarnation for the purpose of spiritual evolution. The material world is considered to be the training ground for souls. As they evolve and reach higher dimensions above the seventh dimension – or the world of angels – they begin to act as guiding spirits.

## 2. Religion and Infection

A previous review has already reported that research conducted prior to 2010 examines the relationships between religiosity/spirituality and the susceptibility to infection (Koenig, 2012). *Religiosity* and *spirituality* can be defined broadly as any feelings, thoughts, experiences, and behaviors that arise from a search for the "sacred," with the former implying group or social practices and doctrines, whereas the latter tends to refer to personal experiences and beliefs (Hill, 2000). Herein, nine out of thirteen studies (69%) have shown that religiosity/spirituality is associated with lower rates of infection or a lower viral load, while none found a greater susceptibility to infection. The findings from several of these studies could be explained by differences in sexual behavior. However, the capacity to prospectively predict lower rates of periodontitis, a lower susceptibility to meningococcal infection, lower viral loads in human immunodeficiency virus-positive patients, and lower death rates from infection/sepsis in stem cell transplant patients does support the notion that religiosity/spirituality involvement may help to protect against infection, and could be as a result of better immune function (see the discussion concerning some possible mechanisms in section "6. Possible mechanisms").

More recently and comprehensively, Hummer and colleagues (Rogers et al., 2010) analyzed data from a sixteen-year prospective study of a national representative sample consisting of 22,080 non-institutionalized adults over the age of 18. Participants completed the baseline survey in 1987, and mortality data were collected through to 2002. To date, this is the largest U.S. national cohort prospectively followed in order to examine the effects of religious attendance on infectious mortality. Controlled covariates and/or cofounders were: demographics (age, gender, race, and region), social ties (marital status, social activity, friends to count on, and relatives to count on), socioeconomic status (education and income), health behaviors (cigarette smoking, alcohol use, and body mass index), and health status (activity limitations, self-reported health, and bed days). Investigators note that controlling for health status at baseline produces a conservative estimate of the effect, given that these health characteristics may have already been affected by religious attendance before 1987.

In terms of religious attendance (an independent variable in the study), a much greater proportion of females frequently attend religious services, despite the observation that similar proportions of males and females never attend religious services. Among those who attend religious services more than once per week, only 35% are male. Compared to white Americans and non-Southerners, relatively more African-Americans and Southerners attend religious services on a more frequent basis. Those who attend religious services more frequently are more likely to be married than unmarried, to be more socially active, to have friends and relatives that they can count on, to abstain from drinking alcohol, and to have never smoked. For example, 41% of those who have never attended religious services are current smokers, whereas only 11% of frequent attendees of religious services are current smokers.

Finally, 20,139 cases remained for the purpose of analysis; of this number, 86 were identified as having died due to infectious disease (all-cause decedents = 3,934) between 1987 and 2002. Controlling for demographics, social ties, socioeconomic status, health behaviors, and health status, non-attendees exhibited 2.15 times (HR = 2.15, $p < 0.05$) greater risk of infectious disease mortality as those who attended services at least once a week. More interestingly, the same comparison, when made along the lines of sex between non-attendees and those who attended religious services at least once a week, reveals that females who do not attend services at least once a week had a much higher risk of infectious disease mortality (HR = 3.80, $p < 0.05$) than males who similarly did not attend services regularly (HR = 1.22, not significant). Regarding infectious diseases, the data suggests that females tend to receive greater resistance from frequent church attendance.

# 3. Prayer in Happy Science

## 3.1. The Theory of Happy Science Prayer

One of the major religious activities is prayer, which has been classified as the most widely used of all complementary therapies – particularly when the focus is on promoting overall good health and well-being (Tippens et al., 2009). The term "complementary" derives from the broader term "complementary and alternative medicine (CAM)" and refers to forms of treatment used in addition to standard or conventional therapies. This is distinct from "alternative medicine," in which conventional therapies are disregarded and replaced outright by alternative modalities alone.

Indeed, Master Ryuho Okawa has drawn attention to the complementary relationships that can, and do, exist between modern medicine and religion, publishing indications such as that which follows (Okawa, 2008a):

> "How should we understand the relationship between modern medicine and religion? This is a challenging issue. I do believe that modern medicine is guided by divine spirits. Here, let us call the angels of light in the field of medicine 'Gods of Medicine.' When you trace the roots of the Gods of Medicine, you will eventually discover the god Hermes*. Eastern medicine sometimes conflicts with Western medicine, originating in the classic philosophies of Lao-tzu and Chuang-tzu, and Buddhism. There are many past examples in which monks taught medicine. The divine spirits also provide ample guidance to religions that heal people's illnesses. From time to time, the divine spirits perform miracles to deepen people's faith. So, what is important is the cooperation and collaboration between medicine and religion. Physicians with religious faith should be able to heal more illnesses by effectively using

---

* Hermes: A God believed to have resided in Greece 4,300 years ago. Hermes brought prosperity to the Mediterranean area and laid the foundations of Western civilization. Well-known as the god of commerce, prosperity, the arts, travel, and communications, among other endeavours, Hermes is also the God of Healing. The Staff of Kerykeion (also known as the Caduceus Staff), which Hermes is often seen holding, is used even today as a symbol of medical institutions worldwide.

> the power of the mind. They should be able to miraculously cure even the most-deadly illnesses by combining positive words and medicine. Likewise, people of religion should be capable of expanding the number of souls they save by cooperating with the positive side of medicine. The goal is people's happiness; therefore, cooperation is ideal."

Although prayer in Happy Science is shown in detail in another review (Kurokawa et al., 2015), we would like to briefly summarize it here. When one prays, a response is received from the guiding spirits of a particular spiritual group, as defined by one's religious affiliation. For example, Christian guiding spirits hear a Christian prayer. Thus, it can be said that spiritual affiliation is one of the conditions for a prayer to be effective. Spiritual affiliation is defined by one's faith. By the same token, Happy Science is blessed by a large number of guiding spirits who provide support and guidance to Happy Science believers. The question arises as to whether prayers made by nonbelievers have any effect. There are always a number of spirits who may recognize prayers made by nonbelievers, but it is uncertain whether a response could ever be expected from them and, if so, which type of spirit could be expected to respond.

For Happy Science Faithful, the spirit world is the world of thought, and thought is the form of existence of souls in the spirit world. Since the three-dimensional world is a uniquely material world, our physical existence is not compatible with the form of existence in the spirit world. However, thought is communicated between these two worlds. Prayer, in essence, can therefore be seen as a form of thought transmission, which is received and responded to by guiding spirits in the spirit world.

Happy Science Doctrine illuminates upon the differences among types of thought and emotion according to the respective frequencies they maintain. Joy, gratitude, anger, and hatred, for instance, are held to have different frequencies. While each thought and emotion has a different frequency, if one repeatedly emits the same sorts of thoughts and emotions, these frequencies develop a certain tendency towards the soul and, subsequently, each soul may come to partake of his/her individual characteristic frequency.

Happy Science further expounds an important law said to be operating in the spirit world. Known as "The Law of Same Wavelengths Attraction," thoughts successfully communicated to the spirit world are said to do so only when there is a "match" in frequencies. As a result, the spirit world is thought of as a huge conglomerate of realms divided by the differentiated wavelengths of collective thoughts. This distinction is held to occur in both vertical and horizontal directions. In the vertical aspect, spirits are divided into dimensions in accordance with their spiritual development; in the horizontal aspect, however, they are divided into homogeneous communities defined by belief, taste, personality, and so on (Okawa, 2012).

In principle, spirits who belong to different dimensions cannot communicate with one another because their frequencies are not compatible. However, thoughts of a living person in the material world can communicate with other dimensions, and the frequency of thoughts determines which dimension or realm they are able to connect with.

As further defined in Happy Science doctrine, frequencies vary between the realms – from the realm of Hell to the ninth dimension. Therefore, if one has a hellish thought, that thought is instantaneously connected to Hell, while a heavenly thought is connected to heaven. People who carry over and maintain a hellish tendency in their thoughts are destined for Hell (which Happy Science maintains is located in a corner of the fourth dimension and which is made up of a collection of multiple realms of different negative frequencies). Therefore, a negative thought connects with a corresponding realm according to the corresponding wavelength. When one's soul is attuned and connected to Hell, what is known as "possession" occurs. In Happy Science, possession is considered to be the cause of problems such as physical and mental illness, as well as misfortune (Okawa, 2008c).

Given that prayers are responded to by guiding spirits who belong to a higher dimension, a prayer, understood as a thought transmission, requires a frequency that is compatible with the guiding spirits' frequency. Therefore, it follows that the quality of thought is considered one of the requisites for prayer to be effective. In general, negative thoughts and wishes – such as curses and egotistic desires – are rejected by guiding spirits, whereas positive prayers – such as expression of an altruistic wish – are likely to be responded to by high-dimensional spirits (Okawa, 2011).

### 3.2. Private Prayer and Ceremonial Prayer (Kigan)

In Happy Science, prayer that is performed in private is distinguished from a prayer performed ceremonially by a designated priest in a designated place. In Japanese, the latter is called "Kigan," which we will refer to here as "ceremonial prayer." Ceremonial prayers are held in the religious facility of Happy Science, where a Happy Science religious professional performs the role of the priest. The priority in Japanese is "Doushi." There are many types of prayers that are only performed during ceremonial prayer sessions. All prayer scripts are divine revelations written down by Master Ryuho Okawa. Each prayer is directed by a guiding spirit or spirits. Believers expect salvation to be received from those guiding spirits.

When one prays privately, supposing that he/she upholds a degree of strong faith and self-help spirit, the prayer's effectiveness is still liable to be affected by his/her state of mind and the condition of the spiritual environment. On the other hand, when a ceremonial prayer is conducted, the state of mind of the priest and the spiritual environment of the prayer room are diligently maintained; therefore, there is more certainty regarding the efficacious results of prayer. As such, even though one has a good faith and self-help spirit, the state of mind and spiritual environment are variables that affect the effectiveness of prayer. In this respect, ceremonial prayers can be said to be more reliable than private prayers.

Moreover, ceremonial prayers are specifically designed for particular purposes, such as overcoming illness, success in business, academic achievement, marriage, and relationships. Guiding spirits who are specialists in each field are assigned to support prayers. However, such specialist spirits are not assigned to each individual at home. The difference between private prayer and ceremonial prayer may be illustrated by an example of someone who seeks legal assistance: Praying privately to request help is compared to tweeting (via Twitter online) in order to seek legal advice, whereas attending a ceremonial prayer is analogous to visiting an attorney's office directly.

Master Okawa explains that the greatest difference between Happy Science and other religions is that Master Ryuho Okawa – who is the incarnation of El Cantare – has first-hand knowledge of guiding spirits. Master Okawa constantly communicates with those spirits as if telephoning them. Because of his extraordinary abilities, he is capable of channeling the full range of spiritual existences, and has published several hundred books that record conversations or interviews that occur during such channeling. Therefore, it is believed that Master Okawa assumes the authority that commands guiding spirits in high dimensions while he remains in this material world. He indicates that this is the source of the spiritual power afforded to ceremonial prayers in Happy Science, and what distinguishes Happy Science from other groups (Okawa, 1997). Happy Science's guiding spirits include spirits from various religious backgrounds – such as Buddhism, Christianity, and Shintoism – as well as many outstanding spirits, including business people, politicians, scientists, academics, and artists – each of whom has made great achievements while living on earth and have returned to higher dimensional realms.

An applicant of a ceremonial prayer writes down his/her wish on a designated form, which is inserted into a special envelope and placed in front of the altar of the prayer room. Applicants make offerings as tokens of gratitude for spiritual support from heaven. The duration of the ceremonial prayer is generally 20 to 30 minutes long, and consists of several stages:

1. Recitation of the Dharma of the Right Mind
2. Giving thanks to El Cantare and the designated guiding spirit
3. Reading aloud the applicant's name (which may or may not occur depending on the type of prayer and location)
4. Recitation of main prayer script
5. Gratitude and Resolution

Prior to the start of the ceremony, applicants are instructed to calm their minds and deepen their concentration. The ceremony is held either individually or collectively. After the ceremony, each applicant receives a special charm designed for each prayer. Applicants retain their charm for one year and bring them back the following year to the same temple where the ritual was performed.

Every person who attends a ceremonial prayer is instructed to have pure faith, gratitude, a self-help spirit and attitude, and to completely entrust the results to the wills of heaven. Regarding the last point, applicants for prayer are also advised to put the wish out of their minds once they have made their request to El Cantare or to the guiding spirits, and to avoid setting any deadline for the prayer's realization or attempting to prescribe the way it should be realized.

Prayer requests are made in many ways. Believers may visit a Shoja and attend a prayer ceremony in person to realize his/her wish. Alternately, a believer unable to attend in person may request that a Shoja perform a ceremonial prayer for them *in absentia*. Likewise, a believer may apply to have a ceremonial prayer conducted for someone other than him/herself. Religious professionals at every Shoja advise that having all parties involved in the prayer attending the ceremony is the most reliable way to ensure a prayer's effectiveness, although those professionals can and often conduct ceremonies and offer intercessory prayers with one or more parties absent.

## 4. A Double-Blind Randomized Controlled Trial by Happy Science Prayer

Scientifically, our research group has recently reported a double-blind randomized clinical trial in which neither the enrolled depressive patients nor those who conducted prayer were informed of the group allocation (Chida, 2017). Additionally, any doctors and nurses involved in patients' treatment were not informed of the treatment assignment. A single researcher carried out this randomization scheme and wrote down a list of the patients in the intervention group (n = 177), which was then placed in a masking envelope. The envelope was then treated with intercessory prayer twice a day (in the morning and in the evening) for 4 weeks (6 days/week); the morning and evening prayer concerned the Prayer for Recovery from Illness ("*Byoki-Heiyu Kigan*" in Japanese) and the Prayer for Exorcising Evil Spirits ("*Akurei-Gekitai Kigan*" in Japanese), respectively, while patients in the control group (n = 187) received usual care, including medication. The Prayer for Recovery from Illness (available from Happy Science) features a ritual called "El Cantare Healing," which involves a specific action. It is believed that, when a believer recites this prayer and performs the ritual, the healing light of El Cantare is sent down to heal illnesses. The power of faith is essential to this practice. If you have a believing heart, you will become one with El Cantare, and light will begin to enter your heart. Faith has the power to overcome the laws of this world. It connects you to higher dimensions and, as a result, provides one the ability to receive healing energy from those dimensions. The Prayer for Exorcising Evil Spirits (available from Happy Science) involves a specific ritual action called "El Cantare Fight." The logic of the exorcism is as follows: when one recites the prayer, he/she is given assistance from El Cantare and guiding spirits, which, together with the "El Cantare Fight" ritual, exerts the power to drive away evil spirits. Participants' mental status was assessed at three points before and after the intervention (immediately after and three months after) using the Center for Epidemiologic Studies Depression scale (CES-D). In an analysis comparing the intervention and control conditions, we adjusted for important confounders – such as diagnosis, illness duration, medication, religious background, smoking, drinking, body mass index, marital status, and education.

A repeated-measures analysis of covariance on CES-D total change score, and the four CES-D subscales change scores (depressive affect, positive affect, somatic complaints, and interpersonal difficulties), show that "interpersonal difficulties" scores were marginally lower in the treatment group than in the control group – both at the post-intervention point and at the three-month follow-up point ($p = 0.11$). Further subgroup analyses of the CES-D's "interpersonal difficulties" change scores show that depressed patients with a score of ≥16 on the CES-D total score ($p = 0.078$) and non-religious patients ($p = 0.079$) tended to show improvements in interpersonal difficulties over the course of the trial. More intriguingly, university graduates (≥16 years of education) exhibited a significant improvement in interpersonal difficulties ($p = 0.007$), both at the point of post-intervention and at the point of a three-month follow-up.

Although this trial failed to confirm that the Happy Science prayer had an ameliorating effect on depressive symptoms in a double-blind randomized controlled trial with Japanese outpatients with depression, power analysis on the actual effect size of approximately 1.2 on the total CES-D suggests that around 2,500 participants (n = 1,250 in each group) would be necessary to confirm the efficacy. Few previous religious interventions have reported any treatment effects on specific CES-D subscales. In this study, the treatment effect appeared to be stronger for interpersonal difficulties than for the other CES-D subscales. If this is a genuine effect, it could be mediated, in part, by interpersonal behavioral pathways. For example, religiosity/spirituality has been related to increased social support and better human relationships (Koenig 2012).

Thus, given that depression has so far been proven to strongly deteriorate a wide range of physical diseases (Koenig 2012), Happy Science prayer would have cured them partially by improving the depressive states of those with physical diseases.

## 5. Anecdotal Cases

The following are cases in which healing prayers proved effective on COVID-19. Two representative case studies are introduced here, each featuring an individual who experienced recovery.

## 5.1. Case 1: A Case of Ms. Annette from the United States (Happy Science, 2020b)

Happy Science started conducting "Prayer for Defeating the Infection of the Novel Coronavirus Originated in China[*1]" in early 2020, and Master Okawa's lecture, titled "How to Strengthen Your Immunity," has been widely attended – both in Japan and beyond – from February at Happy Science branches and temples. A devotee[*2] at the New York temple, Ms. Annette (who lives in the United States), also watched this lecture early in March. In the lecture, Master Okawa said:

- A virus has the same "principle as possession[*3]" and has a connection with "fear." Before the virus circulates, "fear" spreads first.
- "Think bright and constructive thoughts," and "Have right faith" – these mental attitudes will strengthen your immunity and can provide the power needed to win against the virus.
- Attain the power of light and spiritual power of Buddha or God.

Master has taught his followers many ways to strengthen one's immunity from a religious and physical perspective. Ms. Annette also learned the mindset of defeating COVID-19 by listening to the lecture.

A few weeks later, Ms. Annette received a call from her mother saying, "I'm having trouble breathing." Listening to her mother's symptoms, she thought he mother might have been infected with COVID-19. Seeing her irritated with her symptoms, Ms. Annette strongly recommended her to go to the hospital and have it checked, as she had a bad feeling. Subsequently, Ms. Annette decided to take "Prayer for Defeating the Infection of Novel Coronavirus Originated in China" and immediately called the Happy Science branch and reserved the ritual

---

[*1] A Happy Science ritual prayer that has a strong power to protect yourself and your loved ones from COVID-19.

[*2] A follower of Happy Science who has devoted to the Three Treasures, which is to have devotion to Buddha, Dharma and Sanga.

[*3] A situation where a living human is influenced by some kind of spirit.

prayer. Ms. Annette herself took the ritual prayer on behalf of her mother. When she attended the prayer ceremony, she felt an immense light. From the bottom of her heart, she was convinced that her mother would be alright.

Ms. Annette then took her mother to the hospital for the checkup, but the doctor told them that it would take a day for the results, with her mother needing to stay overnight at the hospital. The next morning, Ms. Annette received a call from the hospital: her mother had tested "positive."

> "Despite taking the prayer…Why?"

Ms. Annette became worried. When she headed to the hospital, her mother's symptoms were worse than expected. Her mother could breathe only a little with her own power, so she had to use a ventilator to supply oxygen to her lungs. She was in a critical condition and had to be moved to the ward along with other serious case patients. Usually, those wards are completely isolated, but at this hospital, they permitted family members to visit, which meant that those patients assigned to that ward were very "close to death." Ms. Annette was convinced that her mother would be okay because of the ritual prayer, but she was shocked by her mother's condition and she could not hold back her tears.

However, Ms. Annette recalled what she pledged and wrote in the prayer form: "I will throw away all the negativity that I had felt towards my mother. Please let my mother recover." She made up her mind to abandon any ill feelings towards her: "My mother will definitely be okay. My prayers are heard by God. I will do anything that I can to support her." Ms. Annette recalled the blessings that she felt in the prayer ceremony and strongly told herself to believe in them. She regained her calm mind and became constructive once more. In the lecture "How to Strengthen Your Immunity" she remembered that infections have a close relation with "fear," as follows:

- Viruses follow the same principle of possession; thus, "fear" attracts what you are scared of. Therefore, if you have the opposite

mindset of "fear" – like a bright, cheerful, and constructive way of thinking – your power of immunity improves and will be able to cure illness.
- If the family members know this and believe this, even if the person does not know how to strengthen their immunity, it can also promote a strong attitude in the fight against illness.

Ms. Annette's mother was in a critical condition. Her mother was close to 70 years old, and she had asthma and diabetes, as well as feeling emotionally unstable; as such, her power of immunity was low and her power to fight against the virus was weak. Ms. Annette then realized that her mother was seized with anxiety and fear. She tried to encourage her mother to discard her negative feelings. From that day, she had to refrain from visiting because of the hospital's restrictions; however, she never stopped encouraging her mother through phone calls.

With her practice of love, her mother started to regain her calmness. Her mother's way of thinking changed to a strong will, exclaiming: "I want to get out of the hospital as soon as I can." Her ability to breathe on her own increased. Four days after her mother had tested positive, Ms. Annette received a call from the hospital. She was told that her mother was headed to recovery and that she could move back to her original ward. A few days later, the doctor informed Ms. Annette that "She [her mother] will be discharged from the hospital tomorrow." Although her mother had been infected with COVID-19 and was moved to the ward for those in a critical condition, she experienced a quick recovery and was discharged from the hospital within a week or so.

## 5.2. Case 2: Mr. Tony's Case from the United Kingdom (Happy Science, 2020c)

As the situation in the UK was growing more serious because of the wide spread of COVID-19, Mr. Tony was planning to leave the country.

While packing his bags at night, he got an unexpected phone call from his sister. She said that, over the past week, she had been ill and had been experiencing very high fever, shivering at night or while sleeping, aching muscles, and a severe persistent cough. She was convinced that she had caught COVID-19, but Mr. Tony did not know what to say to her because he was leaving the very next day. Although he was in a conflict with what he should do and how he could help her, he told her to call the emergency services and go to the hospital.

Early the next day, as he was ready to leave, he ran to the London Temple of Happy Science and left a note saying, "Please can you conduct a Kigan of 'Prayer for Defeating the Infection of Novel Coronavirus Originated in China' for my sister because it is an emergency and I have to depart from London." So at the airport, he contacted his family in Tokyo and he said, "Please let her know that we are praying for her we are offering our prayers for her and just please make sure she is okay, because I am boarding my flight."

In Tokyo, Mr. Tony heard the news that people were praying for his sister. By performing Kigan not only in London but in Japan as well, many people were praying for his sister and for her quick recovery. He then called her and found that her condition was much better and that the most severe flu-like symptoms had already passed. He was so relieved that she had almost recovered. He definitely followed the following critical factors, as were pointed out in the lecture on "How to Strengthen Your Immunity":

- The power of faith in God works as an immune system. This is one of the reasons that faith can heal illness, and it has been true since ages. Faith strengthens and boosts our immunity.
- Therefore, if we have fear and disregard our faith, our immunity becomes very weak. Too much self-pity will also attract evil things to us, so we should keep it minimal.
- Some people might not believe in what Master Okawa teaches in how to strengthen one's immunity. However, if their family and friends know and believe this, it will be effective. If the follower in the family thinks "His problem lies with this," or "She needs to

change in this way," it will gradually work, and the person's attitude against the illness will become stronger. It will be "Out with the demons, in with good fortune." Therefore, the more people know of this, the better it is.

# 6. Possible Mechanisms

## 6.1. Happy Science's Perspective on the Relationship between Mind and Body

To illustrate the process by which illness is cured by means of prayer, we explain Happy Science's perspective on the relationship between mind and body (Chida, 2015). In Happy Science, the true nature of the physical body is likened to a flowing stream; every cell in our body is constantly in the process of being replaced. Our bone matter changes with the passage of time; every part of our body is continuously being renewed. Not only are we not the same now as when we were born, but we are still in the process of changing. Every day, new cells are being born, while old ones die. Hair, scalp, eyes, nose, mouth, arms, legs, and even our internal organs undergo changes on a daily, moment-by-moment basis, like a flowing river (Okawa, 2008d).

How can we maintain our identity amidst this constantly changing body? It is in fact our mind that defines a self-image that creates our physical state. For example, if we want to strengthen our muscles, we can make them stronger by working out. However, the determination, or thought form, to strengthen our muscles by training them must come first. The same can happen in internal organs as well. For example, if we are trying to live a healthy life to overcome our visceral problems, our condition will gradually improve. However, if you have negative thoughts, and are continuously thinking, "I am always sick, and I am unhappy. I am dying. I have to live seeking the sympathy of others," these kinds of thoughts will make themselves manifest.

A human being is not just the flesh that we see with our eyes but is actually a multi-structured spiritual being temporarily residing in the physical body. The far outer layer of this spiritual structure is called the "astral body." In actuality, the astral body has exactly the same shape as a human being, with eyes, nose, eyebrows, heart, liver, kidney, and other essential organs. A spiritual being with exactly the same shape resides in the physical body. In line with this theory of a multi-structured spiritual being, early Egyptians also believed that a person consisted of a physical body ("khat") and a soul. The soul consisted of three parts: "ka," "ba," and "akh." The "ka" was thought to be an exact double of the person and was the life force that animated the body, which is quite similar to the concept of the astral body. The "ba" was considered as being separate from the life force (ka) and survived after the body died. Given the right circumstances, the "ka" and "ba" would unite after death to form the "akh." The "akh," in turn, "was the transfigured spirit that survived death and mingled with the gods." The "akh" was thought to survive in the afterlife only if the person had lived a good and worthy life (Wisseman, 2003).

The mind is the main controlling force behind everything. Thoughts create the state of the astral body, which in turn determines the state of the physical body. When negative thoughts – such as anger, hatred, dissatisfaction, excessive desire, pessimism, and a sense of inferiority – become concrete in one's mind, those thoughts form a "thought energy cloud." If these thoughts are only temporary, the negative energy will soon dissipate and vanish. However, when this energy continues to exist for a certain length of time, it materializes and results in some form of illness. Those who suffer from illness have a part in their mind that is afflicted with negativity.

These negative thought clouds prevent spiritual light from entering into one's soul. When these clouds are removed via self-reflection, meditation, and prayer, and the light of God starts to shine into one's soul, he/she will be able to be one with God. When one rebuilds his/her body every day by being one with God, his/her illness can no longer exist.

## 6.2. Happy Science's Theory on Disease

In Happy Science theory, 70-80% of diseases are caused almost exclusively by the state of mind (Okawa, 2008c). Master Ryuho Okawa has, in greater detail, indicated that almost all modern diseases are caused by three factors: what we eat, a lack of exercise, and stress (Okawa, 2008d), indicating that our psychological factors might have a much stronger impact on the etiology and prognosis of illness than any physical, environmental, or genetic factors.

One of the illness-causing psychological factors is our subconscious mind, by which we seek refuge in sickness. The truth is that we cannot heal illness because we do not wish to heal it. We can blame sickness on our feelings of dissatisfaction and disappointment and make excuses for the things we have failed to achieve. In short, all can be forgiven if we are sick. For example, our incompetence can be forgiven if we are sick. If our income is not increasing, this is forgiven if we are sick. If we are not good at raising children, this is forgiven if we are sick. The sick person can be ourselves, our children, other members of our family, and other acquaintances. Anybody can be afflicted. Therefore, we need to understand that it is not just a coincidence, but that in some cases sickness can be a chosen form of escape from our lives. This factor includes our subconscious mind in which we want to be sympathized with and paid more attention to by other people because we feel so unsatisfied with the love received from people when we are in non-illness situations.

Another psychological factor is aggressive emotions directed toward others or, alternately, feelings of remorse. For instance, if we were to look inside the hearts of those who had suffered from cancer, we would almost invariably find them filled with hatred, anger or self-reproach. If we are sick, then we reflect on our own mind. Is there anybody against whom we hold a grudge? Indeed, anger and hostility have recently been reported to be associated with coronary heart disease outcomes in both healthy and coronary heart disease populations (Chida, 2009).

In the case of incurable diseases – such as autoimmune diseases or amyotrophic lateral sclerosis – there are three main causes that carry spiritual significance: (1) possession from evil spirits, (2) karma engraved onto the soul before its birth on earth, and (3) a physical disability consequent to the soul's decision to inspire in others feelings of courage, joy, and a sense of purpose in life (Okawa, 2008c). The first factor – concerning evil-spirits' possession that leads to various illnesses – has long been recognized by both Christianity and Islam. For instance, the Qur'an and Islamic theology refer to humans, angels, and jinni as the three beings – as created by God – who can feel, perceive, and be conscious. Jinni are thought to inhabit the unseen world, and can be either good, bad, or neutral, and may be associated with mental illness (Islam & Campbell, 2012). Bad jinni are probably akin to demons, as they are understood in Christianity.

## 6.3. Spirits Possession and Illness

Possession is a state in which a spirit in Hell, or an earth-bound spirit who fails to depart to the other dimensions, influences the mind of a person in the material world. This occurs because the negative mind of a living person attracts spirits who have the same negative mind – according to The Laws of The Same Wavelengths' Attraction. Suppose a human mind is a radio, and thought is a radio wave; under normal conditions, the radio receives and plays the owner's thoughts. However, when possession occurs, the radio picks up noise or "static," representing the thoughts of other spirits. Possession is, so to speak, a condition whereby negative thoughts are mixed up between a living person and a hellish spirit. As a result, the living person's negative feelings and thoughts are enhanced, and uncontrollable desire and emotion may cause them to ruin their own lives. In the case that one is possessed by a spirit who died with an illness – such as cardiac disease – and began to develop the same symptoms as soon as the possession was removed, the symptoms disappeared. Illnesses such as rheumatism and amyotrophic lateral sclerosis are believed to be caused by spirit possession.

Possession takes place when the wavelengths of your mind are attuned to those of a spirit. There are numerous examples of a negative mind; for instance, an envious mind, a mind that is full of dissatisfaction and complaints, a mind that is always abusing others, hurting people with negative words, a cynical mind, a mind that suffers from a persecution complex – and so on. Those who are susceptible to spiritual possession generally suffer from a persecution complex. They believe that people are always bullying them, that they are being hurt or injured, and that they always lose out. They do not assume responsibility for the awful situation that they are in and continue to blame others. Spirits in Hell find it very easy to approach people like this – people who tend not to take responsibility for their own life.

Another kind of negative mind is an angry mind. People who are always angry – those who are filled with unreasonable rage – will attract spirits from Hell. People who easily lose their temper, who say and do terrible things, who complain, or who have a persecution complex and are always blaming others for their misfortune will be approached by spirits from Hell. There is also the opposite type of mind: people with a low self-image, low self-efficacy, low self-esteem, people who think that they are no good, a complete failure, that they are beyond help, and that they should have never been born will also attract evil spirits.

When illness is caused by possession, medical treatment does not provide the needed solutions; so the possession still needs to be removed. While medicine may remove symptoms, their true cause lies in one's spiritual condition, in which his/her mind is attracting evil spirits like a magnet. Therefore, unless the possession is removed, the symptoms recur repeatedly.

At present, dissociative disorders, and especially dissociative identity disorder (DID) – previously known as multiple personality disorder – are suggested to be strongly affected by spirit possession. The latest international major diagnostic guideline of the international statistical classification of diseases and related health problems, 10$^{th}$ revision (ICD-10), by the World Health Organization (WHO), demonstrates that dissociative (conversion) disorders include "Trance and possession disorders," in which there is a temporary loss of both the sense of personal identity and full awareness of one's surroundings; in some instances the individual acts as if they are taken over by another personality, spirit, deity, or "force" (WHO, 1992). The other major diagnostic guidelines of the Diagnostic and Statistical Manual of Mental Disorders 5$^{th}$ edition (DSM-V), by the American Psychiatric Association (APA), show that diagnostic criteria of DID include the disruption of identity as characterized by two or more distinct personality states which may be described in some cultures as an experience of possession (APA, 2013). Herein, possession-form identities in dissociative identity disorder typically manifest as behaviors that appear as if a "spirit," "supernatural being," or outside person has taken control, such that the individual begins speaking or acting in a distinctly different manner.

One fascinating aspect of DID is the fact that distinct alters often exhibit markedly different symptoms or physiological features (Lock and Collogan, 1986; Beauregard, 2012). Sometimes individuals with DID display allergies in some alters, but not in others. For instance, one of Eve's alters ("Eve White") showed an allergic reaction when she was wearing nylon stockings. Strikingly, Eve's original personality ("Eve White") did not. In another study, one alter was allergic to cats, while the other was not. Additionally, alter egos can respond differently to medications. For instance, a woman who had diabetes needed different amounts of insulin depending on which alter was in charge. Clearly, switches between different spirit possessions can be accompanied by distinct immunological changes, which suggests that evil-spirit possession would develop some infectious diseases.

## 6.4. Effectiveness of Prayer in Infectious Diseases

Master Okawa has described what it is that spreads viruses, such as those causing COVID-19, influenza and the common cold (Okawa, 2008b; Okawa, 2014). Human immunodeficiency virus (HIV) was discovered during the first half of the 1980s, and it is believed that spirits work through this pathogen – the same spirits that, earlier in history, spread the plague (i.e., "Black Death") and cholera. After these diseases were eliminated via advances in medical science, the spirits slowly transformed themselves, eventually reappearing as HIV. Likewise, it is possible that the Ebola virus might have developed from the plague and cholera. In this manner, pathogens are also influenced by spiritual elements. This is why, no matter how much research is done on treatment methods for existing diseases, new diseases continue to appear in rapid succession. Of course, viruses and bacteria are the pathogens causing these diseases, but they, on their own, are not very harmful. It is only when they are manipulated by spirits that they become highly contagious. In addition, like spiritual possession, spirits can cause colds and influenza. In fact, when autumn arrives and the weather cools down, insects die off. At around that point, colds and influenza begin to become more prevalent. It is believed that the spirits of some dead insects that cannot return to the spirit world become wandering souls and gather into swarms, spreading cold and influenza.

As mentioned in another section – section "5. Anecdotal Cases" – a virus does not only have the same principle as possession, but also has a connection to fear. Before the virus circulates the body, fear spreads first. Happy Science prayer, by which higher spiritual power can potentially induce a positive attitude in order to break down fear, acquires immunity strong enough to win against the virus, even the Wuhan Coronavirus.

## REFERENCES

[1] American Psychiatric Association. (2013). *Diagnostic and Statistical Manual of Mental Disorders Fifth Edition* (pp. 292-293). New York, NY: American Psychiatric Publishing.

[2] Beauregard, M. (2012). *Brain Wars: The Scientific Battle Over the Existence of the Mind and the Proof That Change the Way We Live Our Lives* (pp. 102-106). New York, NY: HarperOne.

[3] Chida, Y. (2017). Happy Science Prayer Reduce Interpersonal Difficulties among University Graduates with Depression: A Double-Blind Randomized Controlled Trial. *BOAJ Psychology*, 2, 031.

[4] Chida, Y., Schrempft, S., & Steptoe, A. (2016). A novel religious/spiritual group psychotherapy reduces depressive symptoms in a randomized clinical trial. *Journal of Religion and Health*, 55, 1495-1506.

[5] Chida, Y. (2015). *Religion and Health*. New York, NY: Nova Science Publishers Inc.

[6] Chida, Y. & Kim, Y. (2011). Chapter 10 Development of a Novel Spiritual Group Psychotherapy based on the Fourfold Paths: Happy Science Clinic Group Psychotherapy. In Columbus AM (Ed.) *Advances in Psychology Research Volume 81* (pp. 253-264). New York, NY: Nova Science Publishers Inc.

[7] Chida, Y. & Steptoe, A. (2009). The association of Anger and Hostility with Future Coronary Heart Disease. *Journal of the American College of Cardiology*, 53, 936-946.

[8] Happy Science (2020a). *Happy Science official homepage*. July 7, 2020. Available from: http://happy-science.org.

[9] Happy Science (2020b). *Happy Science official homepage*. July 7, 2020. Available from: (Text version) https://info.happy-science.org/2020/1432/ and (Video version) https://www.youtube.com/watch?v=C1WvP4fZxz4.

[10] Happy Science (2020c). *Happy Science official homepage*. July 7, 2020. Available from: (Video version) https://www.youtube.com/watch?v=a6ZtYqIMzSU.

[11] Hill, P. C., Pargament, K. I., Hood, R. W., McCullough, M. E., Swyers, J. P., Larson, D. B., Zinnbauer, B. J. (2000). Conceptualizing religion and spirituality: Points of commonality, points of departure. *Journal of the Theory of Social Behavior*, 30, 51-77.

[12] Islam, F. & Campbell, R. A. (2012). "Satan has afflicted me!" Jinn-possession and mental illness in the Qur'an. *Journal of Religion and Health*, 53, 229-243.

[13] Koenig, H. (2012). *Handbook of Religion and Health 2nd edition.* New York, NY: Oxford University Press.

[14] Kurokawa, H., Matsumoto, Y., Imai, J., Anderson, T. S., Chida, Y. (2015). Chapter 8 The Curative Power of Prayer: Happy Science Doctrine and the Theoretical and Theological base for Prayer-based Health Interventisons. In A. M. Columbus (Ed.) *Advances in Psychology Research. Volume 104.* (pp. 129-154). New York, NY: Nova Science Publishers Inc.

[15] Lock, S. E., Colligan, D. (1986). *The Healer Within* (p. 54). New York, NY: Plume.

[16] Okawa, R. (2014). *The Healing Power* (pp. 181-228). Tokyo, Japan: IRH Press Co., Ltd. (Available only in Japanese and published with the Japanese title of "Za Hīringu Pawā" in 2014 by IRH Press).

[17] Okawa, R. (2013). *The Laws of the Sun: One Source, One Planet, One People*. Tokyo, Japan: IRH Press Co., Ltd. (Originally published as the Japanese title of "Taiyō no Hō" in 1987 in Japanese by IRH Press Co., Ltd).

[18] Okawa, R. (2012). *The Nine Dimensions: Unveiling the Laws of Eternity*. Tokyo, Japan: IRH Press Co., Ltd. (Originally published as the Japanese title of "Eien no Hō" in 1987 in Japanese by IRH Press Co., Ltd).

[19] Okawa, R. (2011). *The Origin of Love: On the Beauty of Compassion* (pp. 24-31). Tokyo, Japan: IRH Press Co., Ltd. (Originally published as the Japanese title of "Ai no Genten" in 2001 in Japanese by IRH Press Co., Ltd).

[20] Okawa, R. (2009). *The Science of Happiness: 10 principles for manifesting your divine nature* (pp. 3-17). Rochester, VT: Destiny Books. (Originally published as the Japanese title of "Kōfuku no Genri" in 1990 in Japanese by IRH Press Co., Ltd).

[21] Okawa, R. (2008a). *Healing Yourself: The True Relationship between Mind and Body* (pp. 222-225). Tokyo, Japan: IRH Press Co., Ltd. (Originally published as the Japanese title of "Kokoro to Karada no Hontō no Kankei" in 2008 in Japanese by IRH Press Co., Ltd).

[22] Okawa, R. (2008b). *My Lover, Cross the Valley of Tears.* (pp. 16-51). Tokyo, Japan: Happy Science. (Originally published as the Japanese title of "Kimi yo Namida no Tani o Watare" in 2008 in Japanese by Happy Science).

[23] Okawa, R. (2008c). *Healing Yourself: The True Relationship between Mind and Body* (pp. 145-156). Tokyo, Japan: IRH Press Co., Ltd.

[24] Okawa, R. (2008d). *Healing Yourself: The True Relationship between Mind and Body* (pp. 207-243). Tokyo, Japan: IRH Press Co., Ltd.

[25] Okawa, R. (2008e). *Healing Yourself: The True Relationship between Mind and Body* (pp. 75-185). Tokyo, Japan: IRH Press Co., Ltd.

[26] Okawa, R. *The true nature of Ceremonial Prayer*. Feb 21, 1997. Available from Happy Science as the Japanese title of "Kigan no Honsitsu" only in Japanese.

[27] Rogers, R. G., Krueger, P. M., Hummer, R. A. (2010). Chapter 15 Religious attendance and cause-specric mortality in the United States. In C. G. Ellison and R. A. Hummer (Eds.) *The Science of Happiness: 10 principles for manifesting your divine nature Religion Families and Health* (pp. 292-320). New Vrunswick, NJ: Rutgers University Press.

[28] Tippens, K., Marsman, K., & Zwickey, H. (2009). Is prayer a CAM? *Journal of Alternative and Complementary Medicine*, 15, 435-438.

[29] World Health Organization. (1992). *The ICD-10 Classification of Mental and Behavioural Disorders* (pp. 156-157). Geneva, Switzerland: World Health Organization.

[30] Wisseman, S. U. (2003). *The Virtual Mummy*. Champaigne, IL: University of Illinois Press.

In: Psychotherapy
Editor: Hayley Boyd

ISBN: 978-1-53618-877-6


*Chapter 5*

# PSYCHOTHERAPY AND POLITICAL AWARENESS: FROM PAST HERITAGE TO PRESENT CHALLENGES

*Nissim Avissar**
Kibbutzim College of Education, Tel-Aviv, Israel

## ABSTRACT

In this article I review major historical psychoanalytic approaches to psychotherapy that had manifestly addressed political issues. In other words, I wish to portray the political heritage of psychotherapy, a lost or forgotten one. Contrary to views considering psychotherapy and politics to be antagonistic to one another, these approaches acknowledged the psychopolitical connection. I believe that this political narrative of psychotherapy is important in the renewal of psychotherapy at present time. The current era is characterized by rapid changes that are bound to affect politics, societies and individuals. These processes of change demand a re-examination of the goals, objectives and methods of psychotherapy. They call for a paradigm shift that may lead to re-inclusion of broad political issues in the psychotherapeutic discourse. I

* Corresponding Author's E-mail: nissimav@gmail.com.

will argue that in the present historical context, the integration between psychotherapy and politics is necessary.

**Keywords:** diversity, history, politics, psychoanalysis, psychopolitics, psychotherapy

## INTRODUCTION

Politics, in the narrow and common sense of the word, refers to governance, state related processes, public representatives, and governmental decision making. This is why "politics, most people assume, takes place only in specifically designed institutions, such as the cabinet, parliament, parties, and the judiciary, which all have to do with the state and the practice of government" (Brunner, 1995, p.xxxiii). This is politics in the limited sense, a narrow and divisive politics. Psychotherapists may well be avoiding just that meaning of the term, that of factional, party politics which does not allow creating closeness and trust and will only lead to arid political wrangling and argument. However, by wholly giving up on the notion of politics they also lose out on some meanings of it that are vital to therapeutic work, indeed, some would say meanings that are right at the center of that work.

Politics in the more expansive sense of the word addresses relations between human beings and the way one person's actions affect those of others. Political action, that is, is bound to be the action of an individual who is not a public figure; in fact such action may well not at all take place in the public domain. Politics in this sense is an aspect of all social relations (Stoker, 1995). We are, nevertheless, dealing here with relations that affect an other, relations of power, whether explicit or implicit. So here the definition of politics closely implicates power, much as it was proposed by David Cooper one of the major figures in the anti-psychiatry movement (whose name he actually coined), "politics has to do with the deployment of power in or between social entities" (Cooper, 1974, p. 4).

In this broader definition, politics is concerned with power relations, with issues of influence, and oppression of an individual or individuals. The connection between this definition of politics and psychological work – with groups, families or individuals – seems obvious, as there are no relationships that are not inscribed by power. And hence the political is about relationships, and those that affect people, their development and well-being.

## THE LAST TABOO OF PSYCHOTHERAPY?

For a long time politics was considered off limits by mainstream psychotherapy. So generations of therapists were instructed to keep away from any visible public activity, especially those that might give away their political affinities. Such avoidance, however, of direct involvement in politics in the narrow sense is only a small aspect of a much wider ranging phenomenon. Even in therapeutic practice and theory very little attention was devoted to how broad political factors (such as ethnicity, gender, or class) affect mental well-being and to how to refer to any political issues that might emerge in the course of therapy. Training and supervision processes have led many therapists to ignore or remove themselves from any realistic response to issues unrelated to the individual and his or her personal associations. Personal characteristics with a political interface were considered largely irrelevant to psychoanalytical techniques and were thus treated in the same interpretative manner as any other subject matter. This is how their political nature and impact was denied and removed.

So for many psychotherapists in the mainstream we can say that politics was a denied aspect of human relations for a long time. As is the case with denials, though the meaning of things was conscious, the attitude was marked by scorn or rejection either of their existence or their importance. Indeed, political narratives of psychology have always been there as long as the discipline has existed without finding their way into the central therapeutic discourse. This is why the notion of politics, along with its associated contents, was excluded, an issue not to be discussed in the context of therapy (including training and supervision), and this is why it is hard to recognize it as such in therapy. Again, the question arises: Why is it here, of all places, that therapy professionals are helpless and anxious? And hasn't the time come to re-examine the influence of what has been called "the last taboo" in psychotherapy (Altman et al., 2006)?

## LEARNING FROM THE PAST TO TRANSFORM THE FUTURE

In view of the current rapid social and cultural changes (that have been accelerated in the current Corona virus pandemic), I believe it to be very apposite to revisit psychotherapy: its tools and activities. I would like to argue that professional-political approaches like the ones described above are bound to play a major role in the renewal of psychotherapy. Right now it is hard to predict how the above described social changes will affect psychotherapy. Still, one channel may include fundamental change in the way psychotherapeutic conceptions and tools relate to the individual's everyday reality, and the annulment of the sharp distinction between the internal and the external worlds. The current cultural revolution, in other words, is bound to lead to the renewed inclusion of politics in the therapeutic discourse and to a focusing on the political aspects of both personal and professional experience.

The history of psychology as a profession is riddled with examples of psychologists or psychotherapists who acknowledged the psychopolitical connection. They examined this connection in their writings, thought of their professional work as a type of political involvement, or considered their political involvement an aspect of their professional work. In this article I present a historical review of psychotherapeutic approaches, pointing out connections between the political context and the nature of a specific psychotherapeutic theory. Following this review I will discuss the possible value of political awareness in psychotherapy at present time.

## SIGMUND FREUD

Early expressions of this combined, psychopolitical view can be found in Freud. As Stein (2003) has noted, Freud's dreams, as they are presented in *The Interpretation of Dreams*, are replete with political subject matter. But even more so, at times – and in contrast with his express reservation concerning psychoanalysts' engagement with politics - Freud comes up with clearly political arguments. By the later stages of World War I, Freud seems to have become a more political person, devoting more space in his writing to social-political issues. This is when he writes (Freud, 1955) the following paragraph, relating to "a situation which belongs to the future – one that will seem fantastic to many of you" (p. 166):

> "At present we can do nothing for the wider social strata, who suffer extremely seriously from neuroses. […] On the other hand, it is possible to foresee that at some time or other the conscience of society will awake and remind it that the poor men should have just as much right to assistance for his mind as he now has to the life-saving help offered by surgery […] When this happens, institutions or out-patient clinics will be started, to which analytically trained physicians will be appointed […] such treatment will be free." (p. 167)

This is Freud's dream of psychoanalysis for the masses, offering a general outline of what might be done to either help or entirely free the poor from their predicament by psychoanalytical means. This is a political statement.

Here individual healing is seen as a contribution to society, and many psychoanalysts felt an obligation to join the ranks. As Elizabeth Danto mentions in her book *Freud's Free Clinics* (2005), it was such contributions, in the beginning, that enabled the establishment of free clinics. The first of these was financed by Max Eitington who would later establish the Psychoanalytic Society in Palestine. The Berlin free clinic opened its doors in 1920, another started in Vienna in 1922, and two more clinics followed in 1926, one in London and one near Berlin. In 1929,

Ferenczi opened a free clinic in Budapest, and more free clinics were opened later in Zagreb, Moscow, Frankfurt, New York, Trieste, and Paris. Danto comments:

> They were free clinics literally and metaphorically: they freed people of their destructive neuroses and, like the municipal schools and universities in Europe, they were free of charge. In the heady climate of progressivism and social movements between the two world wars, psychoanalysis was supposed to share in the transformation of civil society [...] psychoanalysts believed they had a social obligation to donate a portion of their time to the people who could not otherwise afford psychoanalysis. (p.3)

## SECOND GENERATION OF PSYCHOANALYSTS

Even if Freud's own politicization in the wake of World War One remains an unresolved question, there's no doubt about the politicization of the psychoanalytic movement in those years. The 'second generation' of psychoanalysts – those born around 1900 – experienced the ineradicable horrors of war as children or adolescents, as their personalities were being formed. As Russell Jacoby (1983) argued, the second generation rather than thinking of psychoanalysis in the narrow sense as a therapeutic approach took it as a more comprehensive social project. And so a large proportion of the members of the Psychoanalytic Society in Vienna, and even more so in Berlin, in the 1920s and the 1930s, were political activists. This was definitely not a marginal phenomenon: these people formed the mainstream of psychoanalysis. Jacoby claims that most psychoanalysts during this period were socialists or Marxists. Among these political psychoanalysts two men stood out: Wilhelm Reich and Otto Fenichel, who were the leaders of a group also known as "the left Freudians". These two psychoanalysts shared the assumption that his or her surroundings have a serious impact on the individual's mental development and health. This led them to the conclusion that action for social change is not only possible but necessary if the quality of the lives of individuals in society is to be improved and their mental suffering to be ameliorated. They led the Marxist opposition in the Psychoanalytic Society and were committed to both disciplines – psychoanalysis and Marxism – which they considered to be intertwined and complementary.

In his book *The Repression of Psychoanalysis* (1983) Jacoby was the first to reveal a hitherto unknown chapter in the history of psychoanalysis. A group of politically outspoken psychoanalysts, under the leadership of Otto Fenichel, formed in opposition to Freud's declared political neutrality, his avoidance of political commitment or position taking, and his policy of restraint in the face of the rise of Nazism. Fenichel expressed his opinions in favor of political-social change (which he believed to be necessary if psychotherapy was to be successful), both in writing and in lectures, and he did not conceal his communist leanings. He talked about psychoanalysis' social implications, as well as about the relations between socialism and communism on the one hand, and psychoanalysis on the other. But once the Nazis rose to power in 1933, and as the situation grew more personally dangerous, these activities went underground and became totally covert. Now, like Freud before him, Fenichel too lay low in hopes of better times. But unlike Freud, he did not shut up or forbear. He initiated a correspondence between six colleagues, continuing the political-psychoanalytical conversation and the left-analytical tradition. Fenichel would send the letters to these colleagues; they sent their responses to him, and he edited them and put them together, then to re-distribute the resulting letter among them. The others were instructed to destroy the letters on reading, which is what most of them indeed did. This activity continued for a period of eleven and a half years: it included 119 letters, covering thousands of printed pages.

As opposed to Fenichel who conducted his protest activity quietly and avoided confrontations, Wilhelm Reich (1970) did not make a secret of his political activity, his anti-fascist ideas or his party-political sympathies. He was a revolutionary who stood up against the establishment (including the psychoanalytical establishment), stuck uncompromisingly to his opinions, and paid a heavy price. He pioneered the attempt to create an association between psychoanalysis and Marxism, suggesting an organized, planned method, both in theoretical and in practical-therapeutical terms (Reich, 1972). He took one of his fundamental assumptions from Freud, namely that it is sexual deprivation, mostly, that causes neurosis. Reich, however, believed that the repression of sexual drives is influenced by historical and political conditions which are subject to change. Reich borrowed another basic assumption from Marx, according to which ideology or false consciousness is a tool of social oppression. He believed that the main vital force, oppressed with extreme brutality by the authoritarian-patriarchal system, is sexuality as well as the ability to express this force and to experience full and satisfactory sexual release. According to Robinson (1969): "the connection between sexual repression and the authoritarian social order was simple and direct: the child who experiences the suppression of his natural sexuality was permanently maimed in his character development; he inevitably became submissive, apprehensive of all authority, and completely incapable of rebellion" (p.50). This type of experience obviously underwrites society's power bases, allowing exploitation and injustice to continue. Together these two basic assumptions led to a central, guiding idea of Reich's: the key to mental health is sexual liberation. This for Reich did not stay limited to an abstract theoretical insight. He set up free public clinics for sexual hygiene offering sexual counseling, anticonception methods, and even abortions – officially illegal – all free of charge. These clinics made psychoanalysis available to the public at large while also raising public consciousness of the sexual reforms that would need to accompany the revolution (Robinson, 1969).

## POST WORLD WAR II (AMERICA)

The second generation's golden era came to an end with the end of the Second World War. They became refugees, transplanted into new cultures in which they had to change their modes of action and adjust themselves to new conditions. Those who escaped to the United States, especially during the McCarthy period, had reason to be concerned about their status and had to conceal their political past (Jacoby, 1983). This chapter in the history of psychoanalysis has a tragic conclusion, because it was the political psychoanalysts themselves who eventually buried political psychoanalysis: "the political Freudians themselves often facilitated and intensified the repression; this is why it is so difficult to reassemble, even find, the pieces the story. The best sources – the political Freudians themselves – turned silent" (Jacoby, 1983, p. 13). In fact, from the 1950s the political-therapeutic tradition was pushed out of professionals' consciousness, into the margins of professional practice and discourse. As mentioned, this exclusion of the political from the therapeutic discourse must also be understood in a broad historical-political context, especially as the by-product of the horrors of World War 2 and the political persecution of socialists in the United States. Though political-therapeutic thinking continued in feminist as well as in other professional circles, reference to the political field became a veritable taboo in the mainstream (that is, psychodynamic) therapeutic discourse.

But as Totton (2000) mentions, this did not spell the demise of the tradition. A group of psychoanalysts who called themselves "neo Freudians", the most prominent among them Erich Fromm and Karen Horney, formed an opposition to orthodox US psychoanalysis, creating "a left-wing, humanistic version of psychoanalysis which criticized Freud for his exclusive focus on sexuality and on early infancy, his concept of the death instinct, and his denial of the meaningfulness of social and political reform" (p. 18). Fromm, as is well known, was a member of the Frankfurt School of Social Studies, which gave rise to the Frankfurt School which was deeply indebted to Freud and psychoanalysis. Another famous member of the group was Herbert Marcuse whose special contribution was the link between revolutionary Marxism and psychoanalysis. Though himself not a psychoanalyst, Marcuse – as Frosh (1999) mentions – was an extremely influential author who made a sincere attempt to lay bare Freudian theory's inherent radicalism. This, for instance, is what Marcuse wrote: "psychology, in its inner structure must reveal itself to be political. The psyche appears more and more immediately to be a piece of the social totality, so that individualism is almost synonymous with apathy and even with guilt, but also with the principle of negation, of possible revolution" (1970, p. 1).

## 1960's (Europe)

It would take another two decades before voices promoting psychotherapy's politicization made themselves heard once more. In these years, two movements of protest and criticism (social and professional) and of political involvement unfolded within the therapeutic community: one based in England and the other in France. These were the antipsychiatry movement and Lacanian psychoanalysis. I will now briefly describe these. "Antipsychiatry" actually embraces a variety of figures and approaches, often emerging from very different circumstances, uncoordinated and unrelated. The 1960s saw the development of a wave of criticism against professional structures and foci of authority, and of social-political protest that often overlapped. The antipsychiatry people confronted the status quo, often defiantly and at considerable personal risk. Their criticism was directed beyond psychotherapy, at for instance the authorities, public institutions and leaders.

Two figures in the antipsychiatry movement were especially noteworthy: Ronald Laing and David Cooper. They directed their protest and criticism at the power concentrated in the family, the therapeutic community, and society at large. The personal, here, was perceived as a corollary of society and the power relations that inscribe it. This is what Cooper writes: "there are no personal problems, only political problems" (1980, p. 120). Madness, thus, was seen as a political phenomenon. Laing, Cooper and their friends also seriously criticized the psychiatric establishment's common diagnostic and therapeutic methods. These methods, with their arrogant stereotyping and judgment, do not only fail to solve the problem, they actually perpetuate and entrench it. For psychiatric diagnoses have a power to make things happen: they get internalized and become self-fulfilling prophesies. For Laing, in other words, the observer's position affects the object of observation – it will constitute experience. Hence the medical-organismic approach to human beings interferes with free expression; it is oppressive and violent.

Taking a slightly different direction in France, the protest movement there became mainly associated with the work of Jacques Lacan. Undoubtedly Lacan was pivotal in the awakening of the psychoanalytical community, and of intellectuals in general in France in the 1960s. He himself however did not engage in any open political activity and his opinions were not generally known. It seems they were not particularly leftist (Turkle,1979). The people who made up his intellectual circle, however, were very decidedly leftists: "many in the Lacanian camp entered different radical groupings (Maoists, Trotskysts etc.); as with the early left Freudians, one effect was a new initiative to make analysis more widely available" (Roudinesco, 1990, quoted by Totton 2000, p. 23). Many of them were activists who participated in the student revolt of 1968. Some even turned against Lacan himself: one of them was the Lacanian psychiatrist and psychoanalyst Felix Guattari, who together with Gilles Deleuze, the philosopher, wrote the influential *Anti-Oedipus* in 1972.Guattari had been politically involved from the early stages of his psychoanalytical career, and he became more openly and distinctly engaged in the wake of May 1968 (Totton,2000). He rejected any sharp distinction between individual and society and argued that the personal and public dimensions always tend to fuse (Guattari, 1996). This removal of the distinction between the personal and the political led Guattari to conclude that psychoanalysis – with its focus on the individual and the intra-psychic and its implied power relations – entails social disengagement. When the psyche's energies are drawn away from the social domain it loses its vitality and desire. In other words, psychoanalysis, which comes about through work with middle class bourgeois people, re-creates that same bourgeois position: introverted, alienated, complacent and hollow.

## 1970'S AND 1980'S – FEMINIST PSYCHOTHERAPISTS

In parallel, especially during the 1970s and 1980s, trenchant criticism was coming from feminist therapists to the effect that psychotherapy preserved and entrenched gender based power relations. Feminist therapists took it upon themselves to politicize psychotherapy, eventually evolving psychotherapeutic approaches that claimed to constitute 'political action'. Louise Eichenbaum and Susie Orbach (1982), central figures on the scene of feminist psychotherapy, argued that their interest in female psychology was the direct outcome of their activism in the women's liberation movement. They explained that feminist psychotherapy originated in that movement's consciousness raising groups. This also casts light on the practical similarities between feminist psychotherapy with its various tools and those used by the feminist political activists. Criticism of how gendered power relations were being perpetuated was also leveled against psychological theories and treatments. Feminist psychologists accused the discipline of being "a psychology against women", arguing that the psychology establishment was "distorted facts, omitted problems, and perpetuated pseudoscientific data relevant to women" which actually participated in the exploitation of women by means of labeling them, by suppressing them through medication, by sexually harassing them in therapy, by forcibly hospitalizing them, and so on (Wilkinson, 1997).

Feminist therapists adopted the women's movement argument that personal life is a political issue and so psychological aspects of female identity came to occupy a key position in feminists' social criticism. So, for instance, Juliet Mitchell begins the final chapter of her seminal work *Psychoanalysis and Feminism* (1974), a chapter entitled "The Cultural Revolution", by questioning the status of the biological foundation of gender identity, on which Freud tried to base his psychological theories. Boys and girls, argues Mitchell, are born identical but society, from the moment they're born, destines them for different roles. And so the cultural perception of the categories of femininity and masculinity is responsible for both the formation of gender identities and their (social, indirect) oppression. The implication of this is that in order to address the oppression of women and its psychological consequences, there is a need for an all-out social revolution which will change patriarchy's social order. Mitchell in fact politicizes personal identity, promoting a kind of socialist-feminist revolution which will achieve psychological change through cultural change.

Nancy Chodorow in *Feminism and Psychoanalytic Theory* (1989) dedicates the first chapter of this book to a discussion of cross-cultural research which "there are no absolute personality differences between men and women" (p. 23). Personal identity, for Chodorow, is entailed by social and familial structures. This is a statement that holds for the differences between individuals and groups over and beyond gender differences, especially between power sites and minority or disadvantaged groups. It is therefore only natural that these two traditions, cross-culturalism and feminism, are closely related. Indeed, ever since the 1980s the main site of psychopolitical activity in the international discourse on therapy is the one relating to cultural, ethnic-race, class and other types of difference.

## LATE 1980'S AND ONWARD

From the late 1980s this process of repression of the political gradually began to fade. The professional literature began to feature publications referring to the broader political factors affecting psychotherapeutic work or factors that are, vice versa, affected by it. The question thus arises what could it have been in the 1980s that offered the basis for this increasing openness to issues considered anathema until then. Why did this change happen at this particular point in time? At least two answers are possible. One relates to developments in the discursive field of the profession, the other to the global-political situation. These two are also clearly connected. Professionally speaking, the 1980s are the decade in which Intersubjective and Relational theories (Atwood and Stolorow, 1984; Greenberg and Mitchell, 1983) emerged. From this point on, the impact of these approaches on the psychotherapeutic discourse grew markedly. Countertransference and, at a later stage, self-disclosure, came to be seen as legitimate therapeutic phenomena, deserving close scrutiny. The way is very short from here to the inclusion of broad 'political' issues, relating to both patients and therapists, in the analysis of therapeutic processes. Now the investigation of differences between therapist and patient and their mental realities, also included, for instance, reference to gender, class, cultural background. In global political terms, the 1980s are characterized as a period of momentous change. From persistent tension and a sense of impending threat toward relative quiet and an increasing degree of security. The end of the Cold War, the fall of the Berlin wall, and the end of the war of Afghanistan and the Soviet Union significantly reduced the likelihood of another world war and lessened the nuclear threat. At the same time there were new economic and cultural horizons. In the west, as a result, a new middle class emerged and prospered. *Perestroika* and *glasnost* opened the countries of eastern Europe to the west, leading to unprecedented trade and cultural connections. And so this was a decade of change marked by developing communications, openness to the other, and relative political stability. This political climate, we may argue, offered a fertile ground to developments which had been discussed earlier in the professional field.

As I have shown elsewhere (Avissar, 2005) it was similar political conditions which made it possible, in the history of psychotherapy, for politically-conscious psychological approaches to evolve. On the one hand, that is, an awareness of the cost of war and a degree of discontent with the political status quo, and on the other, a considerable sense of personal security. And indeed, from the late 1980s, expressions of psychotherapists' internal-professional scrutiny and self-analysis became notable. Elsewhere (Avissar, 2016), I have surveyed major texts reflecting the changing perspective of the traditional position regarding politics in this period of time. It seems that since then, psychopolitical discourse became more widespread and influential.

## From Past to Present

And so we have seen that this history of psychotherapy abounds with a variety of examples of psychopolitical thinking and action. This is the forgotten narrative of psychotherapy – and I have only presented a small part of it here. This means that there is no need to create the relation between psychotherapy and politics *ex nihilo*: all it needs is rehabilitation. The rehabilitation of subjugated or silenced knowledge systems may be valuable in terms of the range of possibilities for action and experience or the freedom of individuals and groups (White and Epston, 1990). The same goes here: the process of delegitimization of the political in the discourse of therapy and the reintroduction of forgotten sources of knowledge will mean greater space of movement and maneuvering for psychotherapists.

As mentioned, politics which represents power relations, assumes the existence of asymmetric relations which impact both identity and well-being. Once we recognize the political nature of identity, as well as the political nature of psychotherapy, a complex examination becomes possible of the interrelations that contributed to the formation of identity in the past and to the constitution of perceptions (of self and the of the world) in the present. Omitting either one side in this equation is likely to result in damage or suffering, either due to the individual's guilt (internal focus) or by turning her or him into a victim (external focus). The political (cultural, social) third may well help us extricate ourselves from this binary model so as to enable an inclusive view of the individual in his or her changing context. I believe that we are at the height of a paradigm revolution and as is the case with every revolution, there will be those who will suffer as a result. But we cannot freeze and not move on. Such stasis, indeed, would be damaging.

## Politically Sensitive Psychotherapy

Right from the first acquaintance and the early stage of gathering information the politically sensitive psychotherapist will pay close attention to the client's social-cultural context. Emphasis is on environmental-realistic information of a kind that might disclose the client's world view. To use Bourdieu's (1995) terms, the initial inquiry will focus on exploring the field. His statement "To understand is first to understand the field with which and against which one has been formed", is particularly relevant here. Understanding the field – including for instance its central figures; the rules and incentives at play, its sanctions – is tantamount to understanding the person. This does not mean an investigation of objective facts but an attempt to unveil the way the world looks from the perspective of the individual who lives in it. At the same time, the client's subjective description of her or his life also reveals their personal interpretation of their reality, that is, their worldview or their personal stance in the social structure. In the course of time, the relevant environmental forces and constraints will come into view, as well as the effort and inner resources they require of the individual. This type of preliminary inquiry will allow the therapist a better understanding of a client's experience in his or her unique context. It is easier, from this position, to see reality from the other person's point of view (ie, to promote a more empathic experience in the therapist) and to avoid taking a blaming attitude of the kind that is based on the fundamental attribution error. Also, this clarification will draw attention to the reciprocities between individuals and their surroundings.

Perhaps the main issue setting apart politically sensitive from not-politically sensitive psychotherapy involves the power relations within the therapy. This is not really surprising as politics, broadly speaking, refers to the uses of power and how it affects individuals and groups. It is therefore only natural that this issue should be a crucial one in therapy. Totton (2006) suggests that power and the struggle over it play a major role in psychotherapy, and zooms in on the battle between therapist and client over the definition of reality. Thus, in lieu of a discourse revolving around the question "Who is right?", or worse: instead of the therapist's abuse of power in an attempt to gain the upper hand in matters of reality and its interpretation (sometimes in response to the client's demand for him or her to take a position of authority), Totton proposes that therapists approach their clients from a position of equal rights and acknowledge the fact that the therapeutic encounter is almost as daunting to them as it is to their clients.

In matters of interaction and power-relations, a moral-political discussion is particularly to the point. It may prove especially useful to explore dilemmas that come up in the therapeutic conversation because these usually indicate areas of vagueness in the personal experience or point at an unresolved inner conflict. But unlike in the case of unconscious inner conflict, here conflict emerges in the context of the relationship which itself is subject to inquiry as a moral position always arises vis a vis some reality. It may happen that dilemmas do not announce themselves explicitly. Here is an example: Saul is a 42 years old client, a formerly ultra-orthodox man, married with three children. He and his wife have a hard time making ends meet. Following a dispute with his work place and feeling that he was unjustly treated he looked for legal advice claiming several thousand Israeli shekels. In terms of his family's finances, this was no mean sum. Legal advice came up with a quick solution that jarred with common legal practice in this type of case. In a conversation we had, Saul remarked that he felt "a little uncomfortable but OK" with this advice. He said this casually at the beginning of our meeting, in the course of recounting the events of the previous week. This uncomfortableness caught my attention and I decided to take pause, even though the client himself rather made light of the matter. I did mention that I wasn't sure where this clarification would take us, and that it would be all right not to go into it, but Saul took me up on the offer. I tried to find out the details of the objective situation and, simultaneously, what was driving him in all this. This evolved into a moral discussion which carried some risk. It would have been relatively easy to consider my role in this as moralistic – I was aware of this and tried for it not to happen. Saul talked about being dissatisfied with this "shady deal", something with which he was familiar from other situations. He came up with some examples and soon enough more connections to various aspects of his life, past and present, emerged. We entered a long conversation about the values of the orthodox religious world he had left behind, some of which values which he was missing now. He felt that this was the "bitter pill" he had to swallow as a result of the generally worthwhile transition he had chosen to make. We discussed the possible implications of ignoring this dimension of his identity in the long term. Throughout the conversation I kept returning to the image of the bitter pill which might leave residues inside which, eventually, would be painful. In this sense, I said, therapy might offer him an occasion to stop and consider how he would like to live his life and what values he wanted it to be based on. Gradually his need for partnership and belonging in the secular world came into view, his wish for a place where there is mutual help and concern for the other. At a later stage I mentioned the politics of his psyche and its democratic inclination ("in the worst sense of the word," I added and he raised an eyebrow). I explained the difference between 'ordinary democracy', which is based on the principle of majority rule, and 'deep democracy' which is pluralistic and in which all voices are respected[1]. In the latter case, minorities too are heard and make an impact. This is true for the general political case but also in the realm of the personal. For when certain aspects of our identity (like values, even not the most important ones) are consistently neglected, there is likely to be an accumulation of for instance resentment and bitterness. At the same time we also spoke of the option of making a different choice and to act from non-ethical considerations, that is, the choice to 'cut corners' in the moral domain. Our shared feeling toward the end of this meeting was that what had initially appeared merely a background noise turned out to be a key, defining component of his identity.

In other cases, the political contents may be more narrow and explicit. I believe that political statements are a way of relating to the context in which the individual lives and they express a powerful motivating force. This force could be seen as an expression of care and concern for the environment and community of which the person is a part. Statements of this kind may be consonant with our moral mindset, as therapists and in general, but they may reflect a different perception or even run counter to

---

[1] I borrow this notion from Arnold Mindell's process oriented psychology, especially the part that is dedicated to what he calls 'Worldwork' (Reiss, 2004).

our beliefs. Typical expressions of political materials may relate to certain population groups, whether in an appreciative or a derogatory manner (including, in extreme cases, racist, sexist statements and so on); references to the client's political or social activity, which might involve protest activity; expressions of sadness or pain following certain events, or mention of political discussion in which the client was involved. The obviously most difficult situations are those where there is a gap or even a clash between client's and therapist's views, or between personal therapy objectives and the collective interest, as the therapist sees it. An extreme illustration of this occurred when a colleague told about a young client who was in a bad psychological condition which led him to become very passive and helpless. One of the therapy's main aims was to encourage initiative and activity in his everyday life. This client happened to be someone with radical views and he had even been a member of a militant group in the past. Now the therapist was stuck: the more empowered the client became through therapy, the more he returned to this activity – an activity to which the therapist was squarely opposed and which may offend others. The therapist felt trapped: as though he had to choose between his own worldview and values and the client's well-being. It seems to me that therapeutic work done in a conceptual mode which perceives the individual in her or his context, as part of a collective that is, and is characterized by moral (critical, not dogmatic) transparency would probably have reduced the intensity of the conflict the therapist experienced. These features could among other things have supported the distinction between the client's life and choices and those of the therapist, thus allowing the latter more space and freedom of thought and action.

## ACTIVISM AS PSYCHOTHERAPY

Simultaneously advancing personal change, such a professional position may contribute to social and political transformation and help revitalize politics (Samuels, 2001; Lees & Cleminson, 2015). Here personal psychotherapy situates personal misery in social-political context, hence transforming it into a social or political concern. But there are other, less conventional possibilities as well. Eder (2015) argues that social or political activism is a form of "empathy in action" and views it as a natural extension of therapeutic work. The author states that "it is beneficial for our patients to know we are concerned citizens, actively engaged in our community, and that our empathy for them and others leads us to take action. This allows us to model for them what engagement looks like and gives them permission to become active participants in their communities in whatever way works best" (p. 385). And so the therapeutic has come to be considered inseparable from the political while political action constitutes a main channel for therapeutic intervention.

In his A New Therapy for Politics (2015) Andrew Samuels describes his work in "political clinics" that are "large group events, often composed of people who have nothing to do with therapy and psychology at all, but who come together to explore their emotional and feeling-based reactions to major political themes such as terrorism, the Middle East, racism, homelessness, surveillance" (p. 3). Through this work people often times find out that they have more political interest, knowledge and desire than they imagined. I believe that such a professional stance may serve individuals, groups and societies in this age of political pessimism and demoralization, and help rehabilitate a sense of efficacy and optimism. Research into the relations between activism and well-being support the notion that activism is bound to increase individuals' happiness and their ability to cope with socio-political threats (Boehnke & Wong, 2011; Klar & Kasser, 2006).

A position that makes room for social-political context, moreover, will help the client evolve a sense of the external factors of his or her suffering. This will reduce feelings of failure and guilt and encourage a pro-active attitude. An opening for initiative and action in external reality will thus come about (for both therapist and client, together and each separately), with the objective to introduce change. While these things are bound to make a significant social contribution to the community they also offer a source of personal satisfaction and self-worth deriving from the act of giving and from feeling that one manages to live a meaningful life in an oppressive reality.

## Conclusion

Psychotherapy, facing contemporary challenges, can (and in fact should) take on a more significant social or political role. In this Corona virus era, when gaps widen and hardship become more prevalent, psychotherapists can assume the role of the flag-bearer of an ethics which may support every person's right to live well in conditions of basic security – both physical and mental. If this is what they want to achieve, psychotherapists will have to clarify and redefine their values – to clarify what kind of relations they want to entertain with political domains. They will have to consider what types of power are at play in the reality in which they operate and to situate themselves in this field while keeping constant track of their own actions and their effects. If one takes a clear and uncompromising position this also requires dealing with the disagreement of, and conflict with, those who subscribe to a clashing approach. This may well lead to real struggle and criticism, from within and without. In my opinion, this is a necessary condition for change.

## References

Avissar, N. (2016). *Psychotherapy, Society and Politics: From Theory to Practice.* New York, NY: Palgrave-Macmillan.

Avissar N. (2005). A Community in Conflict: Therapists React to Reality. *Analiza Irgunit*, 9, 25-41 [Hebrew].

Altman N. (1995). *The Analyst in the Inner City: Race, Class, and Culture through a Psychoanalytic Lens*, Hillsdale. NJ: The Analytic Press.

Altman, N., Benjamin, J., Jacobs, T. & Wachtel, P. (2006), Is Politics the Last Taboo in Psychoanalysis?. In: Layton L., Hollander N. C. and

Gutwill S. (Eds.), *Psychoanalysis, Class and Politics: Encounters in the Clinical Setting* (pp. 166-194). New York, NY: Routledge.

Atwood G. E. and Stolorow R. D. (1984). *Structures of Subjectivity: Explorations in Psychoanalytic Phenomenology*. Hillsdale, NJ: The Analytic Press.

Boehnke, K., and Wong, B. (2011), Adolescent political activism and long-term happiness: A 21-year old longitudinal study on the development of micro- and macrosocial worries. *Personality and Social Psychology Bulletin*, *37* (3), 435-447.

Bourdieu P. (1995), *Sociology in Question*. London: Sage.

Brunner J. (1995), *Freud and the Politics of psychoanalysis*, Cambridge, MA: Basil Blackwell.

Chodorow, N. (1989). *Feminism and Psychoanalytic Theory*. New Haven, CN: Yale University Press.

Cooper D. (1974), *The Grammar of Living*. New York, NY: Pantheon Books.

Cooper D. (1980), *The Language of Madness*, Harmondsworth: Penguin.

Cushman P. (1990). Why the Self is Empty: Toward a Historically Situated Psychology. *American psychologist*, *45* (5), 599-611.

Danto E. A. (2005). *Freud's Free Clinics: Psychoanalysis and Social Justice, 1918-1938*. New York, NY: Columbia University Press.

Deleuze, G., Guattari, F. (1977). *Anti-Oedipus: Capitalism and Schizophrenia*, Minneapolis. MN: University of Minnesota Press.

Eder S. L. (2015), Off the Couch and into the Streets: Psychotherapy and Political Activism. *Smith College Studies in Social Work*, *85* (4), 373-386.

Eichenbaum L. and Orbach S. (1982). *Outside In... Inside Out – Women Psychology: A Feminist Psychoanalytic Approach*. New York, NY: Penguin Books.

*Freud* S. (1955). *Lines of advance in psycho-analytic therapy*. Standard Edition 17.

Greenberg J. R. and Mitchell S. A. (1983). *Object Relations in Psychoanalytic Theory*. London: Harvard University Press.

Guattari, P. F. (1996). *The Guattari Reader*. Oxford, UK, Blackwell.

Frosh S. (1999). *The Politics of Psychoanalysis: An Introduction to Freudian and Post-Freudian Theory* (second edition). New York, NY: New York University press.

Jacoby R. (1983). *The Repression of Psychoanalysis: Otto Fenichel and the Political Freudians*. Chicago, IL: The University of Chicago Press.

Klar M., Kasser T. (2009), Some Benefits of Being an Activist: Measuring Activism and Its Role in Psychological Well-Being. *Political Psychology*, *30* (5), 755-777.

Lees J. & Cleminson R. (2015), Retrieving the Past for a Usable Present: Anarchism, Psychoanalysis and Revolutionary Transformation in the Early 20th Century. *Psychotherapy and Politics International*, *13* (2), 141-153.

Marcuse H. (1970). *Five Lectures*. Boston, MA: Beacon Press.

Mitchell J. (1974). *Psychoanalysis and Feminism: A Radical Reassessment of Psychoanalysis*. New York, NY: Penguin Books.

Reich W. (1970). *The mass psychology of Fascism*. London: Souvenir Press.

Reich, W. (1972). *Sex-Pol: Essays, 1929-1934*. New York, NY: Vintage Books.

Reiss G. (2004). *Beyond war and peace in the Arab Israeli conflict*. Eugene, OR: Changing Worlds Publications.

Robinson P. A. (1969). *The Freudian Left: Wilhelm Reich, Geza Roheim, Herbert Marcuze*. New York, NY: Harper & Row Publications.

Samuels A. (2001), *Politics on the Couch: Citizenship and the Internal Life*. New York, NY: Karnac books.

Samuels A. (2015), *A New Therapy for Politics?*. New York, NY: Karnac books.

Stein Y. (2003). *The Flutist from Vienna*. Jerusalem: Keter Publishing House [Hebrew].

Stoker G. (1995). Introduction. In D. Marsh and G. Stoker (Eds.), *Theory and Methods in Political Science* (pp. 1-20). London: Macmillan Press.

Totton N. (2000). *Psychotherapy and Politics*. London: Sage publications.

Turkle S. (1979). *Psychoanalytic Politics: Jacque Lacan and Freud's French Revolution*. London, Burnett Books.

Whachtel P. L. (1989). *The Poverty of Affluence: A Psychological Portrait of the American Way of Life*. New York, NY: Free Press.

White M. & Epston D. (1990). *Narrative Means to Therapeutic Ends*. London: Norton.

Wilkinson S. (1997). Feminist Psychology. In: Fox D. R. and Prilleltensky I. (Eds.), *Critical Psychology: An Introduction*. Beverly Hills, CA: Sage.

In: Psychotherapy
Editor: Hayley Boyd

ISBN: 978-1-53618-877-6


*Chapter 6*

# SHAME IN THE CONTEXT OF DOMESTIC VIOLENCE

***Silke Schwarz****
Wandlitz, Brandenburg, Germany

## ABSTRACT

Contextualizing phenomena requires accounting for specifics that evolve over history, such as locally specific morals and values and culture-specific frameworks for sense-making of people`s experiences, as well as political and institutionalized structures. The discipline of psychology usually evokes a division between the individual and her or his sociocultural context as well as between the mind and the body. This double division is rooted in a particular conception of the subject, the self, and emotions, which is prevalent in Western thinking; this conception separates inner experience and outside expression and implies a culture of individuality and interiority (Taylor, 1989; Zaumseil & Schwarz, 2014). By this, the discipline of psychology risks becoming an apolitical approach which helps to reproduce existing power structures by silencing and pathologizing those who are most in need. This article uses insights from the discipline of psychology on shame and its relatedness to

* Corresponding Author's E-mail: silke.schwarz@fu-berlin.de.

aggression and puts them into the contexts of domestic violence and political structures from a critical and feminist standpoint. Shame is used as an analytic tool for the interconnectedness between private experience and a socially structuring moral realm. The shame experience of men as well as that of women in domestic violence contexts is discussed.

**Keywords:** shame, aggression, domestic violence, intimate partner violence, feminism

## Introduction: The Need for Contextualization

The process of contextualizing phenomena requires us to account for certain specific elements that evolve over history, such as locally specific morals and values and culture-specific frameworks for sense-making of people`s experiences, as well as political and institutionalized structures. In a globalized world, we are also embedded in wider settings and contexts. In a feminist approach, this translates into accounting for universal structural patterns of oppression with a simultaneous sensitivity for specific local and individual factors. The discipline of psychology usually evokes a division between the individual and his or her sociocultural context as well as between the mind and the body. This double division is rooted in a particular conception of the subject, the self, and emotions, which is prevalent in Western thinking; this conception separates inner experience and outside expression and implies a culture of individuality and interiority (Taylor, 1989; Zaumseil & Schwarz, 2014). By this, the discipline of psychology risks becoming apolitical thereby reproducing existing power structures by silencing and pathologizing those who are most in need.

In this article, the interweaving of micro and macro dynamics is demonstrated with the example of shame, presenting the inner realm of personally experiencing shame that is common in mainstream psychology, while also embedding shame in the context of intimate partner violence. Shame is read as an analytic for understanding the neatly intertwined nature of the internal and the external – of the private and the socio-political realm. This article starts by presenting the structures of domestic violence and the ways many researchers describe shame in the context of domestic violence, that is, as one of many other barriers to leaving an abusive relationship. The next two sections discuss insights from the psychological literature on shame and the relationship between shame and aggression. The following section again links the personal with the political, allowing us to consider the complexity between micro and macro dynamics. The final section takes a meta-perspective on how the domestic violence literature understands culture and its influence on shame, elaborating on religiously informed understandings of honour-based violence. Overall, the article analyses shame (or honour – usually understood as its opposite) as a mechanism for transmitting a gender hierarchy and maintaining male dominance, which is interwoven with objective economic and social structures that disadvantage women and children.[1]

## Shame in Domestic Violence Contexts

Since the 1970s, feminist movements have increasingly brought the issue of violence against women into public light (Herman, 1993). According to the World Health Organization (2014), about 30% of ever-partnered women throughout the world have experienced physical and/or sexual violence at the hands of an intimate partner at some point in their lives. The prevalence rate ranges from around 23% in high-income countries to around 36% in low-income African countries. It was only in 2004 when the first representative study was made available in Germany, which is one example of an Organisation of Economic Co-Operation and Development country where prevalence research was conducted as recently as the early 21st century. This late onset of research in this topic is

[1] For example, the total gender wage gap in OECD countries amounts to 13.9 percentage points in 2016 (OECD, 2018). The gender wage gap is defined as the difference between median earnings of men and women relative to median earnings of men. Data refer to full-time employees and to self-employed people.

typical for the long tradition of silencing gender-based violence. The German study demonstrated the high levels of violence against women (BMFSFJ, 2004). More than 10,000 women in Germany were interviewed about their experiences of violence at different points in their life (BMFSFJ, 2004). The results indicate that at least one in every four women aged 16 to 85 years old, living with a partner, has experienced physical assault (23%), while 7% had also experienced sexual assaults at least once.

In intimate partnership violence, men are the predominant offenders and women and children the ones affected by violence. The pattern is not random and studies show a gender-based social structure for both the committing and the suffering of violence. While men are also affected, it is not to the same extent or in the same way (WHO, 2014; BMFSFJ, 2004; Senatsverwaltung für Arbeit, Integration und Frauen, n.d.). Most studies regarding domestic violence focus on women. Research suggests that the types of violence committed by women and men vary with health consequences seeming to be gendered, as well (Swan, Gambone, & Caldwell, 2008). Although there is evidence to suggest that male victims also suffer psychological harm through partnership violence, studies find more negative mental health effects for women compared to men (Ehrensaft, Moffitt, & Caspi, 2006; Tjaden & Thoennes, 2000; Anderson, 2002).

A feminist lens with a power-critical foundation helps to understand both the various ways in which power and control are violently exercised as well as shame, guilt, honour, and other barriers to freedom from abuse. Traumatic experiences, such as intimate partner violence, often induce self-focused emotions, like shame, in survivors both in the wake of trauma and in its aftermath (Wilson, Drozdek, & Turkovic, 2006). Researchers consider shame as one emotion among many other factors to hinder help seeking (such as fear of economic deprivation, fear of being hurt or even killed, fear of social isolation etc.). It is worth noting that the extent to which disclosure leads to healing is still controversial (Graham-Bermann, Kulkarni, & Kanukollu, 2011; Lamb & Edgar-Smith, 1994). Disclosure, however, may reduce the risk of further victimization as well as increasing the likelihood that victims will receive the necessary treatment for the psychological and physical health consequences of abuse and that legal interventions will be initiated (Ullman, Starzynski, Long, Mason, & Long, 2008).

The reasons women do not seek help are similar to those of children who are survivors of domestic violence. Lev-Wiesel, Gottfried, Eisikovits, and First (2014) examined factors affecting disclosure among Israeli children in residential care due to domestic violence. The main hampering factors for disclosure were: emotional (e.g., shame: 39.1%); fear of losing social support and resources (e.g., fear that family would be hurt: 35.6%); and not knowing how or to whom to disclose the information (e.g., do not know to whom to tell: 34.9%).

Morgan, Williamson, Hester, Jones, and Feder (2014) conducted a study with male survivors of domestic violence. When men are victims of domestic violence it is also the female (ex)-partners often being the perpetrator. The most important explanation men give for not reporting abuse is the belief the police would not take any action. The interviews revealed a range of reasons why men were ambivalent about seeking support for relationship difficulties and potentially abusive behaviours. In general, they cited, as barriers to help seeking, the private nature of relationships and the difficulties that they experienced (often due to shame or embarrassment) in discussing problems openly. A participant recalled how he avoided asking advice from his male friends as he felt that they would simply tell him to "go out and shag somebody else or go and get drunk and you'll feel better" (Morgan et al., 2014, p. 640). Masculinity—that is, the stereotypical expectations around being a 'man'—and male identity roles are combined with a reluctance to discuss relationship issues and emotional well-being with others. Many of the male participants expressed difficulties in talking to anyone—friend, family or professional—about emotional and 'personal' issues (Morgan et al., 2014). The sociocultural construction of masculinities and femininities is interwoven with personal scopes of agency as well as cultural beliefs of honour and religious piety (see also later `the role of culture in domestic violence contexts`).

A feminist standpoint seeks to understand this interrelatedness between cultural and religious norms, as well as the intertwining of power relations and personal experience. The personal is embedded in broader analytical levels, such as the family, community, or society, and it is inherent in power dynamics. Shame is read as a socially structuring moral order that operates, as Scheff (1988) has shown, as a primary mechanism for conformity as well as "a ferocious attack on the self," as Lewis (1987, p. 7) has pointed out. The latter is the common level of analysis in the discipline of psychology that encompasses the study of behaviour, the mind, feelings, and the inner experiencing per se. A thorough understanding of the micro dynamics of shame is insightful. It informs us about the power of internally experienced ambivalence, of felt isolation, of the challenges to resisting or changing, and about how to approach and work with people in therapeutic contexts. However, the individual-oriented understanding dominant in the discipline of psychology can also blur the social dimension of experiencing shame along with the related health outcomes. Social and cultural aspects may remain on the outside, as moderating factors, and are not addressed in terms that are intermingled with their inner, private, or cognitive aspects (Taylor, 1989; Zaumseil & Schwarz, 2014). This paper exemplifies how a psychological understanding of shame can be embedded in different contexts, that is, into the political structures of the societies in which we live.

## Insights from the Micro Dynamics of Shame

In this section, I explore the dominant approach to shame in psychology by presenting its definition and its relationship with other emotions by reporting existing relevant literature. What behavioural tendencies are linked to the experience of shame? What adaptive and maladaptive trajectories are linked to the experience of shame? What are the links to clinical psychology and mental disorders?

In dominant perspectives of psychology, shame is usually manifested as an excruciating psycho-physiological affect with thoughts of worthlessness and inferiority, as well as an immediate desire to hide, cover up, or transform the feeling (e.g., into anger) to reduce its impact on the self (Nathanson, 1992; Tangney, Wagner, Fletcher, & Gramzow, 1992). Markers of shame are considered relatively universal and innate in much psychological research. Tracy & Matsumoto (2008), for instance, report findings that blind, congenitally blind, and sighted athletes from different nations all express virtually identical expressions of shame. Wurmser (1987) suggests that "the eye is the organ of shame par excellence" (p. 67), and an initial behaviour following shame activation is eye-gaze diversion in the form of lowering the gaze away from the shaming stimuli or from other people (Darwin, 1872/2009; Keltner, 1995). What is problematic with this universal approach in mainstream psychology is its blindness to sociocultural specifics. It fails to acknowledge that the experiencing and expressing of emotions is embedded in meaningful contexts of historically and biographically rooted symbolic patterns. From a sociological perspective, experiencing and expressing shame differs depending on the social structuring of the moral order (Scheff, 1988), which depends on available and specific cultural ideals of masculinity and femininity.

Psychology usually aims to inform us about intra-psychic specifics through the differentiation of state and trait aspects. The acute experience of shame is thus measured as a state of shame. An ongoing proneness to shame is assessed as trait shame, which is understood to reflect enduring thoughts and feelings associated with the self as inferior. From this perspective, individuals who experience frequent feelings of shame may develop trait shame or shame-proneness as a part of their identity, learning to expect shame experiences and to hide their flawed sense of self from others (Harper, 2011).

In everyday language, the terms 'shame' and 'guilt' are often used interchangeably and rather imprecisely. However, theory and empirical studies in psychology indicate that shame and guilt are different emotions. The essential difference lies in whether the individual is negatively evaluating the global self or a specific behaviour (Lewis, 1971). Feelings of guilt are experienced when an individual's focus is on his or her behaviour – for example, "I did that horrible thing." Feelings of guilt are often accompanied by feelings of remorse and regret. Individuals are likely to become preoccupied with the specific transgression, often wishing they could undo the action. Thus, in mainstream psychology, guilt often motivates one towards reparation, confession, or apology (Fee & Tangney, 2012). Shame, on the other hand, involves a focus on the self as defective or unworthy, beyond the specifics of the behaviour – for example, "I'm a horrible person." This negative evaluation is often associated with a sense of shrinking and feeling small, as well as a desire to hide or disappear. These feelings of shame are much more comprehensive and seemingly inescapable than the specific feelings about a behavioural characteristic of guilt (Fee & Tangney, 2012).

In mainstream psychology, the process of coping with this privately understood shame experience can be summarized by Nathanson's (1992) shame model, which, in turn, encapsulates observations from many shame theorists. His model includes four shame-regulation strategies: attack self, attack others, withdrawal and avoidance. 'Attack self' involves internalization, self-directed anger, and even disgust. 'Attack other' involves externalization of blame and anger, and even aggression. 'Withdrawal' involves internalization and attempts to reduce social exposure. 'Avoidance' involves emotional minimization or denial in attempts to keep shame from awareness. In the context of domestic violence, experiencing shame can be linked with self-harming behaviours in female survivors, as well as with a tendency to socially withdraw themselves, leading to isolation. Isolation is also often a consequence of a pattern of control by their abusive partners. Among other factors such as fear of being physically harmed or even killed, shame hinders them from leaving an abusive partner. Many perpetrators also explicitly use shaming strategies as a control instrument, destroying the self-worth and esteem of affected women.

In contrast, men exerting domestic violence may experience shame and transform it into 'attacking others' as well as 'avoidance' of feelings that potentially threaten their masculinity.

This knowledge about micro dynamics helps to understand phenomena that appear to be illogical from the outside (e.g., why a woman stays with her abusive partner) and can inform clinical practice about what needs to be detangled. 'Suppression' and 'avoidancc' present one of the greatest challenges for clinicians and researchers as shame becomes hidden from the individual experiencing it (Garfinkle, 2012) and, thus, from health professionals who care for them. Jurist (2005) argued that alexithymia (i.e., the inability to identify and describe emotions in the self) as a construct may be useful in investigating the relationship between early traumatic attachment experiences and impulsive aggression. Tangney, Stuewig, Mashek, & Hastings (2011) have argued that alexithymia involves the inability to identify painful feelings of shame, as those shamed would be inclined to defensively externalize blame outward onto a convenient scapegoat. These linkages between shame and aggression are discussed in the next session, which focuses on interactions in violent contexts.

In general, shame serves both negative and positive psychological functions. For instance, shame plays an adaptive role in motivating and regulating people's thoughts, feelings, and behaviours, as well as in driving "people to work hard in achievement and task domains [...], or to behave in moral, socially appropriate ways in their social interactions and intimate relationships" (Tracy & Robins, 2007, p. 4). It translates into a moral order opposing domestic violence. The moral orders differ across sociocultural contexts and the section on `The role of culture in domestic violence contexts` below explores this issue.

By contrast, shame also acts in a maladaptive way by mediating the negative emotional and physical health consequences of social stigma (Feiring, Taska, & Lewis, 2002), or by way of its association with a wide range of personality pathologies, emotional disorders, and psychiatric diseases according to mainstream psychology (Tracy & Robins, 2007). Research indicates that shame has a significant association with general stress reactions (Pinto-Gouveia & Matos, 2011) and with post-traumatic stress disorder (PTSD), especially when the trauma exposure includes high levels of emotional and verbal abuse and experiences of subordination and isolation (Beck, McNiff, Clapp, Olsen, Avery, & Hagewood, 2011). These insights called for the provision of counselling services for domestic violence survivors, in order to help them cope with the atrocities they had to experience. As WHO (2013) has recommended, psychological counselling is needed in women's shelters, as is routine sensitization training of medical staff in the health sector to equip them with knowledge of the relationship between intimate partner violence and mental health.

Because guilt results from specific behaviour, one may assume that it exerts a lesser psychological toll than shame, as with shame the person evaluates their entire self as negative. To date, guilt has received more attention in the trauma literature than shame. However, Beck and colleagues (2011) found in their study with women experiencing domestic violence that shame correlated significantly with PTSD severity, while guilt did not show an association. In one set of studies, traumatic memories about shaming experiences amplified the intensity of depression (Matos & Pinto-Gouveia, 2010) and served as a significant predictor of paranoid ideation and dissociation (Matos, Pinto-Gouveia, & Duarte, 2012). Without diminishing the importance of fear and anxiety in understanding PTSD, numerous authors have recognized the role of other forms of negative emotion, particularly shame, guilt, anger, and sadness (e.g., Brewin, Andrews, & Rose, 2000; Lee, Scragg, & Turner, 2001; Pitman, Orr, Forgue, Altmann, de Jong, & Herz,1990). These emotional states may shape how PTSD symptoms are presented, the extent to which an individual responds to exposure-based treatments, and whether further treatment is needed following exposure. Furthermore, Rhatigan, Shorey, and Nathanson (2011) showed that post-traumatic symptoms, such as PTSD and depressive symptoms, shame, and reduced self-efficacy, may be risk factors for remaining committed to and involved with violent partners over time, thereby potentially increasing the risk of continued abuse.

## INSIGHTS FROM THE MICRO DYNAMICS OF AGGRESSION AND SHAME

As noted above, shame can serve as a trigger for violent acts (Walker & Knauer, 2011). This supports the relevance of shame and aggression as useful focus for clinical interventions aimed at perpetrators of intimate partner violence (Lawrence & Taft, 2013). From an evolutionary perspective in mainstream psychology, shame is considered as a basic emotion family (e.g., feelings of inferiority, embarrassment, humiliation) elicited by perceptions of negative evaluations by others of characteristics or actions that one attributes to one's self, causing social pain (Velotti, Elison, & Garofalo, 2014). MacDonald and Leary (2005) theorised that social pain co-opts the mechanisms of physical pain and, thus, of physical threat-defence mechanisms (i.e., fight-or-flight). The threat-defence mechanism of physical pain must often be rapid and automatic, operating prior to conscious evaluation, and sometimes operating as a panic response. As a result, shame—as with physical pain—may result in maladaptive defensive aggression, even against innocent others. If shame leaves one feeling weak and inferior, anger may restore one's sense of worth, control, and power. Threats to self-esteem can trigger aggression. The link between shame and aggression has been observed in partner violence, incarcerated violent offenders, and personality disorders (Narcissistic, Borderline, Antisocial), with shame acting as a common antecedent to violence (Velotti et al., 2014). It is important to note that shame as triggering of rapid and automatic intimate partner violence is not equated with loss of control per se. Perpetrators usually act violently in order to restore their self-esteem; it is an instrumental and rational behaviour. They seldom act spontaneously, but rather, they commit the assault in private and leave marks on their victims' body parts that cannot be seen.

With regard to personality features and pathology, Kivisto, Kivisto, Moore, and Rhatigan (2011) found that shame moderated the link between antisocial attitudes and three kinds of partner violence (i.e., physical assault, psychological aggression, and sexual coercion) among men. Research also documents the facilitating role of threatened masculinity (Moore & Stuart, 2004) and attachment insecurity (Sonkin & Dutton, 2003) in batterers.

Tangney and Dearing (2002) argue that shame is characterized by low concern for others and high concern for the self and that shame experiences could heighten emotional distress and self-concern, which, in turn, could result in interpersonal hostility. In a recent review, Walker and Knauer (2011) argued that shame should be considered a key trigger—and self-esteem patterns as key vulnerabilities—for violence. Jones and Elison (2013) investigated shame-focused coping in response to social exclusion, including self-esteem as a moderator. They found a three-way interaction between inclusion–exclusion, sex, and self-esteem when predicting attack or other responses (i.e., externalized blame and anger from Nathanson's 1992 model). There was a main effect in which males with low self-esteem self-reported more attacks of others than males with high self-esteem, regardless of the inclusion/exclusion condition, supporting the view that low self-esteem is a risk factor for aggression. However, males with low self-esteem were less likely to endorse attacking others when excluded as opposed to included, but males with high self-esteem were more likely to attack others when excluded than when included. It appears as though exclusion may have inhibited aggressive responses in low self-esteem males, whereas exclusion increased aggression in high self-esteem males, which is consistent with a social dominance perspective. Females showed a contrasting pattern of responding, in that high self-esteem females endorsed 'attack other' more than low self-esteem females, supporting the opposite view—that high self-esteem is a risk factor for aggression. The interaction between self-esteem and inclusion–exclusion was more pronounced for females. Once again, in contrast to males, females with low self-esteem endorsed 'attack other' more when excluded than when included; females with high self-esteem endorsed 'attack other' more when included. Thus, self-esteem appears to be an important and complex moderator between feelings of exclusion and anger, possibly operating differently for males and females.

Felson and Massoglia (2012) reported that many sexual assaults occur during consensual sexual relations, when the man wants to go further than the woman and uses physical force when she resists. With regard to personality pathologies, sexual refusal is tightly linked to aggression through narcissistic personality features (Bushman, Bonacci, van Dijk, & Baumeister, 2003). Moreover, rejection sensitivity (namely, the disposition to anxiously expect, readily perceive, and react in an exaggerated manner to cues of rejection in the behaviour of others; Downey, Feldman, & Ayduk, 2000) has been found to be useful in predicting aggression among romantic partners (London, Downey, Bonica, & Paltin, 2007). Shame feelings themselves increase the propensity to appraise ambiguous events as representing probable rejection (Claesson & Sohlberg, 2002). In turn, aggressive acts are fostered by both expected and unexpected rejection by peer-groups (Twenge & Campbell, 2003; Wesselmann, Butler, Williams, & Pickett, 2010). Taken as a whole, these findings implicate shame as one of the core emotions operating in those situations that have been documented to predict violent outcomes in relationships. However, gendered hierarchies and power structures of society in which domestic violence occurs are not adequately accounted for in the discipline of psychology.

## Linking the Personal with the Political in a Feminist Clinical Setting

The previous two sections have explored the tendency within psychology to emphasize cognitions, motives, and goals of a person. A division is drawn between the individual and his or her sociocultural context, as well as between the mind and the body. By this, the discipline of psychology risks becoming an apolitical approach which helps to reproduce existing power structures by silencing and pathologizing those who are most in need. Although sociobiological theories emphasize reproductive fitness from an evolutionary perspective, and attachment and psychoanalytic theories emphasize terrifying fears of abandonment, feminist theories emphasize patriarchal entitlement and an unequal distribution of power within our society (Kivisto, 2014).

Gender-based violence should be understood not just as a dynamic between a survivor and a perpetrator on a personal or an interactionist level, which is undoubtedly important, but also between the person and an unequal distribution of power within society (Schwarz, 2017a/b). The psychological (emotions and actions) is inherently social and does not emerge from the inner, individual self. Shame in domestic violence contexts illustrates this. Based on my clinical experience with domestic violence survivors and perpetrators, gendered contexts are invariably reflected in the client's narrative in therapy sessions. In my work with a married Indian woman who had fled her abusive marriage, her narrative included shame and guilt because she felt she had disappointed her parents and the broader community. In this case, her story was interwoven with the social script she had internalised throughout her life within her extended family: that women who go against cultural norms are 'bad.' Shame, as well as sociocultural norms about what it means to be a woman or a man, transmit gendered hierarchies that are interwoven with socioeconomic structures of oppression. The client had to face a life of repudiation and persecution by her family and economic hardship after leaving her abusive marriage.

A male client from Bosnia-Herzegovina came to therapy suffering with flashbacks from experiences in war and 'rage explosions.' The post-war environment, marked by a tight economic situation, led to his unemployment, which contributed to a high level of frustration and inner tension, combined with low self-esteem. He felt ashamed and 'unworthy as a man' due to being unemployed and he felt disrespected by his wife and children. He quickly interpreted their behaviour as a sign that they were not being submissive and respectful enough towards him as the head of the family. This interpretation served as his justification for violent acts against his wife and children. After the police imposed an expulsion order, his wife (and their children) faced economic hardship, communal gossip, harassment, and accusations of failing to maintain domestic harmony.

A context-emphasizing, socio-critical approach encourages work with a client's biography, cultural values and moral codes. It takes the social context and unequal power relations as the starting point, which has implications for the understandings of disease and health, as well as the therapeutic relationship and the applicable psychotherapeutic techniques. The therapeutic task lies in strengthening flexibility in applied coping strategies in order to avoid reinforcing gender stereotypes and therefore gender-based violence (for psychotherapeutic details, see Schwarz, 2017b). A feminist approach is about enabling clients to identify internalised messages and replace them with self-enhancing beliefs while developing a range of behaviours that are freely chosen (Corey, 2005). This is especially integral in working with survivors of gender-based violence because of the impact that the internalising of perpetrators' messages has on the survivor's sense of self.

Besides therapeutic goals (that is, providing relief for the person suffering), feminist work also usually includes political aims—here, the eradication of domestic violence. It involves political engagement that aims to change the contexts in which we live into a more equal distribution of power, generally speaking. Feminist clinical psychologists oscillate between clinical practice and political activism. In the endeavour to erase violence against women, working with the perpetrator has therefore become another important focus alongside working with the survivors (Gahleitner, 2013).

## THE ROLE OF CULTURE IN DOMESTIC VIOLENCE CONTEXTS

A feminist approach also takes a critical stance towards its own discipline, so as to take a meta-perspective and to examine the way in which hegemonic gazes might exclude certain groups and thereby perpetuate existing power structures. Honour-based violence illustrates this. Honour is informed by cultural morals and understood to be the opposite of shame on a family or community level. In an exploratory study of honour crimes in the United States, Hayes, Freilich, and Chermak (2016) point to the importance of honour in strengthening behaviours and the significance of avoiding shame for the family in the context of honour killings. Westernized behaviour, which brought shame upon the family, was used to justify honour killings. Shameful behaviours included dressing in Western attire, wearing make-up, dating or having male friends, resisting a forced marriage, or seeking a divorce (Hayes et al., 2016). Partners were usually the offenders, and the violence often occurred in the course of separation.

While most research on culture and violence focusses on Islamic contexts and highlights the issue of honour killings (Eisner & Ghunheim, 2013; Payton, 2014), Marsden (2014) qualitatively explores the issue of domestic violence in a Christian community. Most of the women interviewed specifically referred to the admonition to forgive 'seventy times seven' and considered this to be a God-given expectation, even in the circumstances of abuse that they faced. Domestic violence was further supported by the tenet of 'forgive and forget' rather than recognising previous abuse and acknowledging they had been sinned against. Above all, patriarchy and complementary gender roles function to keep the women in abusive marriages. The ideal of the submissive female leads to women in traditional marriages, where the husband is considered to be the head of the family, being victimised three hundred per cent more often than women in egalitarian marriages in Christian communities (Marsden, 2014).

The example of honour killings shows that social and cultural scripts may contribute to a perpetuation of existing power structures. In order to understand the role of culture in relation to shame and violence, it is important to deconstruct our biases of viewing culture as the cause of violence, and to be able to view culture from a different lens. Culture includes the beliefs, practices, values, norms, and behaviours that are shared by members of a group. Cultural values and beliefs play a significant role in shaping a woman's experience of abuse and its meaning to her. Cultural factors pertaining to marriage and family honour have a significant impact on women's help seeking (Levy, 2008; Tonsing, 2016). Tonsing (2016) shows that women can be reluctant to seek help or talk openly, as disclosure is seen as dishonouring and as bringing shame to the family. The reasons for this were varied, including concern for their children's well-being and future prospects, fear of being ostracised from the community, and maintaining family honour. Culture also encompasses power structures such as being dependant on the husband. In the case of a divorce, for example, no support from one's own family is to be expected, or one could lose a visa sponsorship via the husband.

A feminist perspective on shame in domestic violence contexts highlights this entanglement of personal experience with the broader cultural, social, economic, and political context. It calls for context-sensitivity instead of individualizing and decontextualizing personal experiences from the sociocultural and economic settings in which they are embedded. Therefore, knowledge about local culture and related values is needed beyond that about shame or domestic violence itself. In a collectivist culture, the individual represents the family. Hence, he or she is expected to protect the honour and prestige of the family, at all times. It is important that secrecy and loyalty be maintained and that no individual deliberately injure the dignity of the family or community. This is to ensure a harmonious life. It is linked to the concept of 'face' often described in reference to the Chinese community, and also found in the Indian and Malay cultures. It involves filtering information that may embarrass or shame the family (Ow & Katz, 1999). Another important aspect of this concept of loyalty is filial piety, derived from Hindu, Buddhist, and Confucian teachings, where the young are taught to respect, obey, and care for their elders. Families find ways to keep the family integrity intact because of the concepts of 'face,' shame, and filial piety. Religious teachings in all cultures also reinforce the ideals of loyalty, honour (Anwar, 1998), and respect for parents (Nair & Osman, 2012). In collectivist cultures, such as Asian backgrounds, women are very reluctant to discuss matters that might attract any negative attention onto themselves or their families. Othman, Goddard, and Piterman (2014) show, in the Malay context, how women would rather suffer personally than bring about public suffering and are more concerned about the well-being of others. Therefore, domestic violence should be resolved by the spouses, not by others. A 'good' wife would not publicly humiliate the family and show the husband's limitations. All of these cultural beliefs hinder help seeking and produce feelings of shame if one breaks with these cultural norms.

The example of honour-based violence also helps to illustrate an ethnocentric bias: Payton (2014) shows that Western feminism plays a dominant role in current approaches to domestic violence. It concentrates on conjugal relationships and neglects extended family relationships. Thereby, domestic violence is located within interpersonal dyadic (mostly heterosexual) relationships. Intimate partner violence becomes understood as the 'normal' form of gender-based violence, presumed to be a-cultural, whereas honour-based violence becomes a facet of a divergent culture. This not only makes the category readily available for xenophobic discourse, but also serves to excuse the failures of states to provide support and protection to victimized persons within minority communities, when their victimization is considered 'cultural' and hence rooted in their 'othered' identities (Koğacioğlu, 2004, 2011). If we talk about honour-based violence, we would need to equate this with jealousy crimes: Sexual jealousy is frequently offered as a motivation for violence against women—but there has never been any attempt to create a separate sub-category of 'jealousy crimes' (Payton, 2014).

## CONCLUSION

A feminist approach seeks to understand the interrelatedness of cultural norms, power relations, and personal experience. It accounts for the unequal access to and control over financial, political, and symbolic resources. The personal is embedded in broader analytical levels, such as the family, community, or society.

This article used the phenomena of shame in the context of domestic violence as an analytic tool for understanding the neatly entwined nature of the internal and the external—of the private and the socio-political realms. A review on shame from a psychological perspective can inform feminist psychological theory and practice. The psychological (emotions and actions), however, needs to be understood as inherently social. Therefore, shame was put into the context of domestic violence, illustrating how a context orientation can be linked to a person's psychological inner realm. Above all, this article has emphasized the need for knowledge about local culture and related values, not just knowledge about shame or domestic violence itself.

Shame and recognition are profoundly psychosocial issues (Frost, 2016). Whether toxic or protective, "shame is a reaction to the absence of approving reciprocity" (Ikonen & Rechardt, 2010, p. 112). This failure by the outer world or domain to respond adequately is the primary source of humiliation and shame. In this sense, public policy interventions and laws designed to erase domestic violence should play a crucial role in dealing with the experience of shame and humiliation in domestic violence contexts.

## FUNDING ACKNOWLEDGMENTS

None.

## CONFLICT OF INTEREST

None.

## REFERENCES


Anderson, K. L. (2002). Perpetrator or victim? Relationships between intimate partner violence and well-being. *Journal of Marriage and Family, 64*, 851–863.

Anwar, M. (1998). *Between cultures: continuity and change in the lives of young Asians*. London: Routledge.

Beck, J. G., McNiff, J., Clapp, J. D., Olsen, S. A., Avery, M. L., & Hagewood, H. (2011). Exploring negative emotion in women experiencing intimate partner violence: shame, guilt, and PTSD. *Behavior Therapy, 42*, 740–750.

Brewin, C. R., Andrews, B., & Rose, S. (2000). Fear, helplessness, and horror in posttraumatic stress disorder: Investigating DSM-IV criterion A2 in victims of violent crime. *Journal of Traumatic Stress, 13*, 499–509.

Bundesministerium für Familie, Senioren, Frauen und Jugend (BMFSFJ). (2004). *Lebenssituation, Sicherheit und Gesundheit von Frauen in Deutschland.* Retrieved from http://www.bmfsfj.de/BMFSFJ/root,did=20560.html. [*Living situation, safety and health of women in Germany.*]

Bushman, B. J., Bonacci, A. M., van Dijk, M., & Baumeister, R. F. (2003). Narcissism, sexual refusal, and aggression: Testing a narcissistic reactance model of sexual coercion. *Journal of Personality and Social Psychology, 84*, 1027–1040.

Claesson, K., & Sohlberg, S. (2002). Internalized shame and early interactions characterized by indifference, abandonment and rejection: Replicated findings. *Clinical Psychology and Psychotherapy, 9*, 277–284.

Corey, G. (2005). *Theory and practice of counselling and psychotherapy*. Belmont, CA: Thomson Brooks/Cole.

Darwin, C. (1872/2009). *The expression of the emotions in man and animals*. London: Penguin.

Downey, G., Feldman, S., & Ayduk, O. (2000). Rejection sensitivity and male violence in romantic relationships. *Personal Relationships, 7*, 45–61.

Ehrensaft, M., Moffitt, T., & Caspi, A. (2006). Is domestic violence followed by an increased risk of psychiatric disorders among women but not among men? A longitudinal cohort study. *American Journal of Psychiatry,* 163, 885–892.

Eisner, M. & Ghuneim, L. (2013). Honor Killing Attitudes Amongst Adolescents in Amman, Jordan. *Aggressive Behaviour, 39*, 405–417.

Fee, R. L., & Tangney, J. P. (2012). Procrastination: a means of avoiding shame or guilt? *Journal of social behavior and personality, 15*, 167–184.

Feiring, C., Taska, L., & Lewis, M. (2002). Adjustment following sexual abuse discovery: the role of shame and attributional style. *Developmental Psychology, 38*, 79–92.

Felson, R. B., & Massoglia, M. (2012). When is violence planned? *Journal of Interpersonal Violence, 27*, 753–774.

Frost, L. (2016) Exploring the concepts of recognition and shame for social work. *Journal of Social Work Practice, 30*, 431—446.

Gahleitner, S. (2013). Genderaspekte in der Behandlung von Patientinnen und Patienten mit komplexen Traumafolgestörungen [Gender aspects in the treatment of patients with complex traumatic disorders]. In M. Sack, U. Sachsse & J. Schellong (Eds.), *Komplexe Traumafolgestörungen. Diagnostik und Behandlung von Folgen schwerer Gewalt und Vernachlässigung* (pp. 394–408). Stuttgart, Germany: Schattauer. [*Complex trauma-related disorders. Diagnosing and treating the consequences of severe violence and neglect*]

Garfinkle, E. (2012). Shame: the hidden resistance. *Canadian Journal of Psychoanalysis, 20*, 44–69.

Graham-Bermann, S. A., Kulkarni, M. R., & Kanukollu, S. (2011). Is disclosure therapeutic for children following exposure to traumatic violence? *Journal of Interpersonal Violence, 26*, 1056–1076.

Harper, J. M. (2011). Regulating and coping with shame. In R. Trnka, K. Balcar, & M. Kuška (Eds.), *Re-constructing emotional spaces: From experience to regulation* (pp. 189–206). Prague, CZ: Prague College of Psychosocial Studies Press.

Herman, J. L. (1993). *Die Narben der Gewalt. Traumatische Erfahrungen verstehen und überwinden*. München, Germany: Kindler. [*The scars of violence. Understanding and overcoming traumatic experiences*]

Ikonen, P., & Rechardt, E. (2010). The origin of shame and its vicissitudes. In P. Ikonen & E. Rechardt (Eds.), *Thanatos, shame, and other essays: On the psychology of destructiveness* (pp. 111–138). London: Karnac.

Jones, T., & Elison, J. (2013). *Coping with exclusion changes over time*. Poster presented at the 25th annual Association for Psychological Science convention, Washington, D.C.

Jurist, E. L. (2005). Mentalized affectivity. *Psychoanalytic Psychology, 22*, 426–444.

Keltner, D. (1995). Signs of appeasement: evidence for the distinct displays of embarrassment, amusement, and shame. *Journal of Personality and Social Psychology, 68*, 441—454.

Kivisto, A. J. (2014). Abandonment and engulfment: a bimodal classification of anxiety in domestic violence perpetrators. *Aggression and Violent Behavior, 19*, 200–206.

Kivisto, A. J., Kivisto, K. L., Moore, T. M., & Rhatigan, D. L. (2011). Antisociality and intimate partner violence: the facilitating role of shame. *Violence and Victims, 26*, 758–773.

Lamb, S., & Edgar-Smith, S. (1994). Aspects of disclosure mediators of outcome of childhood sexual abuse. *Journal of Interpersonal Violence, 9*, 307–326.

Lawrence, A. E., & Taft, C. T. (2013). Shame, posttraumatic stress disorder, and intimate partner violence perpetration. *Aggression and Violent Behavior, 18*, 191–194.

Lee, D. A., Scragg, P., & Turner, S. (2001). The role of shame and guilt in traumatic events: a clinical model of shame-based and guilt-based PTSD. *The British Journal of Medical Psychology, 74*, 451–466.

Lev-Wiesel, R., Gottfried, R., Eisikovits, Z., & First, M. (2014). Factors affecting disclosure among Israeli children in residential care due to domestic violence. *Child Abuse & Neglect, 38*, 618–626.

Levy, B. (2008). *Women and violence*. Berkeley: Seal Press.

Lewis, H. B. (1971). *Shame and guilt in neurosis*. New York: International Universities Press.

Lewis, H. B. (1987). The role of shame in depression over the life span. In M. R. Lansky & A. P. Morrison (Eds.), *The widening scope of shame* (pp. 29–50). Hillsdale, NJ: Analytic Press.

London, B., Downey, G., Bonica, C., & Paltin, I. (2007). Social causes and consequences of rejection sensitivity in adolescents. *Journal of Research in Adolescence, 17*, 481–506.

MacDonald, G., & Leary, M. R. (2005). Why does social exclusion hurt? The relationship between social and physical pain. *Psychological Bulletin, 131*, 202–223.

Marsden, D. (2014). Okay, now you can turn it off. *The New Zealand Journal of Christian Thought and Practice, 21*, 4—13.

Matos, M., & Pinto-Gouveia, J. (2010). Shame as a traumatic memory. *Clinical Psychology and Psychotherapy*, *17*, 299–312.

Matos, M., Pinto-Gouveia, J., & Duarte, C. (2012). Above and beyond emotional valence: The unique contribution of central and traumatic shame memories to psychopathology vulnerability. *Memory, 20*, 461–477.

Moore, T. M., & Stuart, G. L. (2004). Effects of masculine gender role stress on men's cognitive, affective, physiological, and aggressive responses to intimate conflict situations. *Psychology of Men and Masculinity*, 5, 132–142.

Morgan, K., Williamson E., Hester, M., Jones, S., Feder, G. (2014). Asking men about domestic violence and abuse in a family medicine context: help seeking and views on the general practitioner role. *Aggression and Violent Behavior, 19*, 637–642.

Nair, S., & Osman, M. M. (2012). Singaporean adolescents' perceptions of violence: implications for practice. *Qualitative Social Work, 12*, 490–506.

Nathanson, D. L. (1992). *Shame and pride: affect, sex, and the birth of the self*. New York, NY: W.W. Norton.

OECD (2018). *Gender wage gap (indicator).* doi: 10.1787/7cee77aa-en (Accessed on 17 October 2018).

Othman, S., Goddard, C., & Piterman, L. (2014). Victims' barriers to discussing domestic violence in clinical consultations: a qualitative enquiry. *Journal of Interpersonal Violence, 29*, 1497–1513.

Ow, R., & Katz, D. (1999). Family secrets and the disclosure of distressful information in Chinese families. *Families in Societies, 80*, 620–628.

Payton, J. (2014). "Honor," collectivity, and agnation: emerging risk factors in "honor"-based violence. *Journal of Interpersonal Violence, 29*, 2863–2883.

Pinto-Gouveia, J., & Matos, M. (2011). Can shame memories become a key to identity? The centrality of shame memories predicts psychopathology. *Applied Cognitive Psychology, 25*, 281–290.

Pitman, R. K., Orr, S. P., Forgue, D. F., Altmann, B., de Jong, J. B., &Herz, L. R. (1990). Psychophysiologic responses to combat imagery of Vietnam veterans with posttraumatic stress disorder versus other anxiety disorders. *Journal of Abnormal Psychology, 99*, 49–54.

Rhatigan, D. L., Shorey, R. C., Nathanson, A. M. (2011). The impact of posttraumatic symptoms on women's commitment to a hypothetical violent relationship: a path analytic test of posttraumatic stress, depression, shame, and self-efficacy on investment model factors. *Psychological Trauma: Theory, Research, Practice, and Policy, 3*, 181–191.

Scheff, T. J. (1988). Shame and conformity: the deference-emotion system. *American Sociological Review, 53*, 395–406.

Schwarz, S. (2017a). Contextualized understandings of health and illness in psychology: the example of domestic violence. *Journal of Social Science & Allied Health Professions*. [Paper submitted, March 2017].

Schwarz, S. (2017b). Psychotherapy in domestic violence contexts. *Community Psychology in Global Perspective, 3*, 1–14.

Senatsverwaltung für Arbeit, Integration und Frauen. (n.d.). *Häusliche Gewalt*. Retrieved from http://www.berlin.de/sen/frauen/keine-gewalt/haeusliche-gewalt/artikel.20187.php. [*Domestic violence*]

Sonkin, D., & Dutton, D. G. (2003). Treating assaultive men from an attachment perspective. *Journal of Aggression, Maltreatment & Trauma, 7*, 105–133.

Swan, S., Gambone, L, Caldwell, J. (2008). A review of research on women`s use of violence with male intimate partners. *Violence and Victims,* 23, 301–314.

Tangney, J. P., Wagner, P., Fletcher, C., & Gramzow, R. (1992). Shamed into anger? The relation of shame and guilt to anger and self-reported aggression. *Journal of Personality and Social Psychology, 62*, 669—675.

Tangney, J. P., & Dearing, R. L. (2002). *Shame and guilt*. New York: Guilford Press.

Tangney, J. P., Stuewig, J., Mashek, D., & Hastings, M. (2011). Assessing jail inmates' proneness to shame and guilt: feeling bad about the behavior or the self? *Criminal Justice and Behavior, 38*, 710–734.

Taylor, C. (1989). *Sources of the self: the making of modern identity*. Cambridge: Harvard University Press.

Tjaden, P., & Thoennes, N. (2000). *Full report of the prevalence, incidence, and consequences of violence against women.* Washington, DC: National Institute of Justice.

Tonsing, J. L. (2016). Domestic violence: intersection of culture, gender and context. *Journal of Immigrant and Minority Health, 18*, 442–446.

Tracy, J. L., & Matsumoto, D. (2008). Spontaneous expression of pride and shame: evidence for biologically innate nonverbal displays. *Proceedings for the National Academy of Sciences, 105*, 11655-11660.

Tracy, J. L., & Robins, R. W. (2007). The nature of pride. In J. L. Tracy, R. W. Robins, & J. P. Tangney (Eds.), *The self-conscious emotions: theory and research* (pp. 263–282). New York: Guilford Press.

Twenge, J. M., & Campbell, W. K. (2003). “Isn't it fun to get the respect that we're going to deserve?” Narcissism, social rejection, and aggression. *Personality and Social Psychology Bulletin, 29*, 261–272.

Ullman, S. E., Starzynski, L. L., Long, S. M., Mason, G. E., & Long, L. M. (2008). Exploring the relationships of women’s sexual assault disclosure, social reactions, and problem drinking. *Journal of Interpersonal Violence, 23*, 1235–1257.

Velotti, P., Elison, J., & Garofalo, G. (2014). Shame and aggression: different trajectories and implications. *Aggression and Violent Behavior, 19*, 454–461.

Walker, J. S., & Knauer, V. (2011). Humiliation, self-esteem and violence. *Journal of Forensic Psychiatry & Psychology, 22*, 724–741.

Wesselmann, E. D., Butler, F. A., Williams, K. D., & Pickett, C. L. (2010). Adding injury to insult: unexpected rejection leads to more aggressive responses. *Aggressive Behavior, 36*, 232–237.

Wilson, J. P., Drozdek, B., & Turkovic, S. (2006). Posttraumatic shame and guilt. *Trauma, Violence, & Abuse, 7,* 122–141.

World Health Organization (WHO) (2013). *Responding to intimate partner violence and sexualviolence against women. WHO clinical and policy guidelines*. Geneva: World Health Organization.

World Health Organization (WHO) (2014). *Global status report on violence prevention*. Geneva: World Health Organization.

Wurmser, L. (1987). Shame: the veiled companion of narcissism. In D. L. Nathanson (Ed.), *The many faces of shame* (pp. 64—92). New York: Guilford Press.

Zaumseil, M., & Schwarz, S. (2014). Understandings of coping: a critical review of coping theories for disaster contexts. In M. Zaumseil, S. Schwarz, M. von Vacano, G. Sullivan, & J. Prawitasari-Hadiyono (Eds.), *Cultural psychology of coping with disasters* (pp. 45–83). New York: Springer.

## About the Author

***Phil Silke Schwarz*** researched on cultural coping mechanisms (book "cultural psychology of coping with disaster") and premarital sexuality in Islamic contexts (book "Selbstbestimmung trotz Tabu?"). As a psychologist she worked for five years in a women`s shelter and now is a scientific consultant to improve health services for domestic violence survivors and their children.

In: Psychotherapy
Editor: Hayley Boyd

ISBN: 978-1-53618-877-6


*Chapter 7*

# HOW IMPORTANT IS PSYCHOTHERAPY FOR BREAST CANCER PATIENTS?

*Cathy-Anne Wendling*[*]
LANSAD Department, University of Strasbourg, Strasbourg, France

## ABSTRACT

The purpose of this chapter is to explore the relevance of psychotherapeutic interventions for female breast cancer patients. Little research has been conducted on the individual perception of the disease and its treatments and of the lack of social support among these patients, though in the last forty years, a growing number of breast cancer autobiographies have been published. This chapter is based on thirty such narratives. These accounts provide crucial information about the psychological experience of the disease and suggest that patients tend to harbor intense negative representations of the illness and the treatment protocol as well as acute feelings of isolation, which may have a detrimental impact on their quality of life, affective states, and immune response. Indeed, long-lasting negative emotions and lack of social support have a harmful influence on individuals' quality of life and level of stress, which in turn can have a toxic influence on the person's mental

[*] Corresponding Author's E-mail: cathy-anne.wendling@unistra.fr.

and physical health. Psychotherapy may help to give rise to less threatening representations of breast cancer and treatment and reduce the patients' subjective perception of loneliness. It can also reduce stress and negative mood as well as improve active coping skills and adherence to treatment.

## INTRODUCTION

From a psychological standpoint, breast cancer is a very distressing experience. This can be observed from the numerous breast cancer autobiographies dealing with the psychological experience of the disease that are being published every year. In fact, written testimonies provide a unique qualitative insight into the psyche of the patients suffering from the disease as they give them an opportunity for the free expression of their emotions, feelings and personal experience; that in turn allows to gain in-depth understanding of their subjective experience. Indeed, the exploration of these accounts has shown that - contrary to what happens during psychological interviews – in written autobiographies, fewer defense mechanisms such as inhibition, repression or suppression bar the access to expressive authenticity. Most women suffering from breast cancer explain that they do not speak about their cognitions and feelings to doctors, psychologists, family, and friends, therefore these aspects of the illness tend to be underestimated or ignored.

## METHOD

Among the three hundred fifty breast cancer autobiographical testimonies I have found on the internet and elsewhere, thirty female patients' testimonials dating from 1975 to 2018 were selected at random in order to explore their representations of the disease and of the cancer treatments as well as their depiction of painful emotions. The authors of those autobiographies are 30 to 65-year-old western American, British and

French women from various social backgrounds. This qualitative study used content analysis. The selection criterion was meaningful occurrences of a detailed description of the subjective representations of breast cancer and cancer treatment as well as the description of negative affect. Narrative and content analysis were used in order to determine the relevant material and the prevalence of the breast cancer and treatment representation theme. Those descriptions, which were found in sixteen breast cancer accounts among the thirty, were extracted and categorized using keywords. Relevant quotations were transcribed and listed, and semantic directories of the patients' linguistic expressions, images, and meaningful metaphors were compiled. Content analysis revealed a repeated pattern among those quotations, which were explicitly associated with intense and prolonged negative emotional states. As a clinical psychologist, my question was whether those representations and feelings may have a negative impact on the patients' quality of life and health status.

## REPRESENTATIONS OF BREAST CANCER

First of all, these narratives indicate that breast cancer tends to give rise to a wide range of deleterious perceptions. According to Anagnostopoulos & Spanea, these representations play an important role in the exaggerated negative perception of the disease[1]. For instance, these authors have noted that women harbor breast cancer representations that are characterized by an underestimation of the illness' curability and an overly negative view of its physical consequences. In fact, Ashley et al. point out that the meanings attached to breast cancer play an important role in the psychological experience of the disease as they tend to impact the

[1] Anagnostopoulos, F. & Spanea, E. (2005). Assessing illness representations of breast cancer: A comparison of patients with healthy and benign controls. *Journal of Psychosomatic Research* 58: 4, 327-334.

patients' affective states, quality of life and their immune functioning in an adverse way[2].

In the autobiographies I have studied, I have found the following individual representations of the occurrence of breast cancer among female patients:

- F. Prevost: 'a monstrous population[3]'
- S. Nethery: 'a roaring lion, a gnawing demon[4]'
- S. De la Brosse: 'a monster inside my body[5]'
- A. Francos: 'a demon', 'a slow death[6]'
- M.A. Sarton: 'roots and tentacles floating on stagnating water[7]'
- B. Maillard-Chaulin: 'a crab[8]'
- K. Russell Rich: 'a gas main exploding', 'a sinkhole[9]', 'a bully[10]', 'a silent stalker, a panther[11]', 'a menagerie of death[12]', 'death inhabiting my bones[13]', 'a greedy pig[14]', 'a lion, wild cats[15]'
- C. Anderson-Copeland: 'something gnawing away at my body[16]', 'a ticking time bomb[17]'
- R. Thomason: 'destructive termites eating my body[18]', 'a death sentence[19]', 'Visigoths deflowering my temple[20]'

---

[2] Ashley, L., Marti, J., Jones, H., Velikova, G. & Wright, P. (2015). Illness perceptions within 6 months of cancer diagnosis are an independent prospective predictor of health-related quality of life 15 months post-diagnosis. *Psycho-oncology* 24 :11, 1463-1470.

[3] Prevost, F. (1975). *Ma Vie en plus.* Paris : Stock, p. 10.

[4] Nethery, S. (1978). *One year and counting: Breast cancer, my world, and me.* Ada, MI : Baker Book House, p. 61.

[5] De La Brosse, S. (1979). *La Force de vaincre.* Paris : Lattès, p. 65.

[6] Francos, A. (1983). *Sauve-toi, Lola.* Paris: Editions Bernard Barrault, p. 113.

[7] Sarton, M.A. (1997). *Recovering.* London: Women's Press, p. 186.

[8] Maillard Chaulin, B. (1999). *Journal d'un sein.* Orléans: Editions Corsaire, p. 189.

[9] Russell Rich, K. (1999). *The Red devil: To hell with cancer.* New York: Crown Publishers, p.16.

[10] Ibid., p. 54.

[11] Ibid., p. 81.

[12] Ibid., p. 127.

[13] Ibid., p. 139.

[14] Ibid., p. 180.

[15] Ibid., p. 204.

[16] Anderson Copeland, C. (2000). *Coming through the darkness.* Springfield, MA: Destiny Press, p. 56.

[17] Ibid., p. 57.

- E. Accad: 'an alien entity[21]', 'the bad cells eating the good ones[22]', 'the 20th century plague[23]', 'masculine aggressiveness[24]', 'a venomous scorpion[25]', 'mad cells trying to kill[26]', 'a sacrifice[27]', 'a fetus between pregnancy and tumor[28]', 'a stalker[29]', 'monsters devouring me, demons[30]', 'mass destruction[31]'
- C. Brunet: 'an attacking bear[32]', 'a bastard[33]'
- F. Rubert: 'a disgusting beast[34]', '9/11, violence[35]', 'terrorism[36]', 'evil[37]'
- G.K. Baker: 'cancer with insidious claws[38]', 'moving in, eating my sternum, throttling my throat[39]', 'a time bomb[40]', 'tainted cells[41]'
- M. Norton: 'an old dog, a bloodthirsty doppelganger[42]', 'a shark[43]'
- M. Vaillant: 'announced death[44]'
- S. Tabet: 'seeing myself dead[45]'

---

[18] Thomason, R. (2000). *Shoring up my soul: A year with cancer*. West Conshohocken, PA: Infinity Publishing, p. 6.
[19] Ibid., p. 16.
[20] Ibid., p. 63.
[21] Accad, E. (2001). *The Wounded breast.* Melbourne: Spinifex, p. 46.
[22] Ibid., p. 70.
[23] Ibid., p. 89.
[24] Ibid., p. 98.
[25] Ibid., p. 147
[26] Ibid., p. 157
[27] Ibid., p. 175.
[28] Ibid., p. 339.
[29] Ibid., p. 349.
[30] Ibid., p. 359.
[31] Ibid., p. 471.
[32] Ibid., p. 128.
[33] Ibid., p. 174.
[34] Rubert F. (2006). *La Vie est là, simplement*. Paris : Albin Michel, p. 14.
[35] Ibid., p. 117.
[36] Ibid., p. 118.
[37] Ibid., p. 124.
[38] Baker, G.K. (2008). *Cancer is a bitch.* Da Capo Lifelong Books, p. 1.
[39] Ibid., p. 14.
[40] Ibid., p. 22.
[41] Ibid., p. 102.
[42] Norton, M. (2008). *Lopsided: How having breast cancer can be really distracting*. New York : Viking, p. 119.
[43] Ibid., p. 191.
[44] Ibid., p. 12.
[45] Tabet, S. (2010). *Les Patientes*. Paris : Les Empêcheurs de penser en rond, p. 103.

The representations mentioned by these authors can be divided into 8 categories:

- Images of threatening animals
- Representations of evil or of an inner enemy
- Fantasies of sexual aggression or rape
- Fantasies related to a monstrous pregnancy
- Images of a rotting substance
- Images of invasive and disgusting vegetation
- Images of war: bombings and terrorist attacks
- Impending death

These negative fantasies tend to give subjective strength to cancer cells and therefore result in pessimistic expectations. For instance, Norton mentions strong, well-shaped, extraordinary cells with huge nuclei and Tabet writes that it would be madness to think that she could be cured. Moreover, the meanings attached to the disease are associated with prolonged and intense negative emotions: Russell Rich mentions depersonalization, Thomason writes about a great feeling of vulnerability and Anderson Copeland experiences intense depression. Accad speaks about her acute fear and Ireland also mentions mind-numbing fear. Brunet notes panic attacks and bottomless depression, Vaillant feels annihilated, and Tabet experiences intense rage. The acute negative contents of the images used by the sixteen quoted patients to describe their illness indicate that despite medical progress and reassuring messages from the medical field, the subjective representations of breast cancer are attached to fantasies of intrusion, violence, and destruction. The quoted autobiographies show that these images tend to be intensely frightening and threatening and that the perception of the illness is associated with intense and lasting negative affective states such as fear (Accad), anger (Tabet), and depression (Anderson Copeland). That may have several harmful consequences. Indeed, the meanings those women attach to the disease are linked to a high level of perceived threat (Nethery, Accad), severity (Francos, Tabet), and uncontrollability (Prevost, De La Brosse).

Freiman-Gibb et al. have also underlined that the emotional representations of breast cancer are significantly correlated with fear of recurrence[46].

These subjective meanings can elicit representations of a fatal incurable illness and have a detrimental impact on compliance with treatment. In fact, according to Linn, Linn & Stein, how a person perceives a particular disease will influence not only health preventive behavior, but also whether medical care will be sought in the face of symptoms and whether the patient will adhere to the treatment protocol[47]. In effect, Ashley et al. have noted that intensely negative illness cognitions are associated with more passive ways of coping. What's more, Rozema, Vollink & Lechner observed that patients who view their disease as uncontrollable report poorer physical and mental health[48]. This is all the more the case as these representations tend to be resistant to change[49].

## REPRESENTATIONS OF THE TREATMENT PROTOCOL

In addition, many subjects mention that their perception of cancer treatments also bring about acute and prolonged negative affect. Indeed, Andersen et al. have observed that radiotherapy gives rise to ongoing anxiety[50] while Knobf has indicated that chemotherapy provokes

[46] Freiman-Gibb, L.A., Janz, N.K., Katapodt, M.C., Zikmund-Fisher, B.J. & Northouse, L. (2016). Illness representations, risk perception, and fear of cancer recurrence in breast cancer survivors. *Psycho-oncology* 26:9.

[47] Linn, M.W., Linn, B.S., & Stein, S.R. (1982). Beliefs about causes of cancer in cancer patients. *Social Science and Medicine*, 16(7), 835-839.

[48] Rozema, H., Vollink, T. & Lechner, L. (2009). The Role of illness representations in coping and health of patients treated for breast cancer. *Psycho-oncology* 18:8, 849-857.

[49] Mc Corry, N.K., Dempster, M., Quinn, J., Hogg, A., Newell, J., Moore, M., Kelly, S. & Kirk, S.J. (2013). Illness perception clusters at diagnosis predict psychological distress among women with breast cancer at 6 months post diagnosis. *Psycho-oncology* 22:3, 692-698.

[50] Andersen, B.L., Karlson, J.A., Anderson, B. & Tewfik, H.H. (1984). Anxiety and cancer treatment: Response to stressful radiotherapy. *Health Psychology* 3, 535-551.

significant distress[51]. Sinsheimer & Holland have reported increased depression and diminished hope in chemotherapy patients[52].

## Representations of Treatments

### Surgery

- Gray: about mastectomy: 'I was expecting to look like a bomb had landed on me[53]'
- Susan: '(we were) the splice girls[54]'. 'this ritual of sacrifice[55]'
- B. Maillard-Chaulin: 'a slaughtering[56]'
- R. Thomason: '(I was) sliced off, scraped out, sewn up, shorn, stripped, scarred for life[57]'
- E. Accad: 'mutilations against women, excision in the name of custom[58]', 'a barbaric practice[59]'
- F. Rubert writes that surgery reminds her of 'Nazi camps and torture[60]'
- G.K. Baker: 'my breast smashed on a tray like a slab of meat[61]', 'pierced with fishing hooks[62]'
- Tootie: 'I feel like I have been gutted like a deer[63]'

---

[51] Knobf, M.T. (1986). Physical and psychologic distress associated with adjuvant chemotherapy in women with breast cancer. *Journal of Clinical Oncology* 4, 678-684.
[52] Sinsheimer, L.M. & Holland, J.C. (1987). Psychological issues in breast cancer. *Seminars in Oncology* 14, 75-82.
[53] Shook, R.L. (1983). *Survivors: Living with cancer*. New York: Harper and Row, p. 22.
[54] Kuner, S., Osborn, C., Quigley, L. & Stroup, K. (1999). *Speak the language of healing: Living with breast cancer without going to war*. Berkeley, CA: Conari Press, p. 187.
[55] Ibid., p. 84.
[56] Maillard Chaulin, B., ibid., p. 27.
[57] Thomason, R., ibid., p. 12.
[58] Accad, E., ibid., p. 156.
[59] Ibid., p. 167.
[60] Rubert F., ibid., p. 56.
[61] Baker, G.K. (2008). *Cancer is a bitch*. Da Capo Lifelong Books, p. 29.
[62] Ibid., p. 30.
[63] Pettason A. *I am not my breast cancer*. New York: Harper, 2008, p. 321.

- M. Vaillant: 'having been violated, violence[64]'

## Chemotherapy

- A. Francos: 'a holocaust[65]'
- B. Joseph: '(chemo) views the body as a war zone[66]', it is 'a demonic torturer[67]'
- K. Russell Rich: 'a rifle[68]'. 'The body is being poisoned[69]'
- R. Thomason: 'pumping in poisons[70]', 'receiving the red devil and the white demon[71]', 'my body was being destroyed, like pesticide that zaps the roach and poisons the dog[72]', 'it has penetrated some of my heart cells, of which it's destroying some[73]'
- C. Anderson Copeland: 'I feel like a woman preparing for the electric chair[74]'
- E. Accad: 'a vicious liquid, which contains so many poisonous elements[75]', 'torture, it's truly torture[76]'. *In a dream*: 'a dog, a biting animal, an intravenous injection of poison.[77]'
- C. Brunet: 'my enemy, a disease[78]'
- F. Rubert: 'machines of death[79]', 'torture[80]'

---

[64] Vaillant, M. (2008). *Une Année singulière avec mon cancer du sein*. Paris: Albin Michel, p. 49.
[65] Francos, A., ibid., p. 89.
[66] Joseph B. *My Healing from breast cancer.* New Canaan, Connecticut: Heats Publishing, 1996, p. 15.
[67] Ibid., p. 57.
[68] Russell Rich K., ibid., p. 204.
[69] Ibid., p. 91.
[70] Thomason, R. (2000). *Shoring up my soul: A year with cancer.* West Conshohocken, PA: Infinity Publishing, p. 42.
[71] Ibid., p. 43.
[72] Ibid., p. 44.
[73] Ibid., p. 503.
[74] Anderson Copeland C., ibid., p. 65.
[75] Accad E., ibid., p. 69.
[76] Ibid., p. 139.
[77] Ibid., p. 393.
[78] Brunet C., ibid., p. 64.
[79] Rubert F., ibid., p. 46.
[80] Ibid., p. 79.

- M. Norton: ‘I became convinced that nobody had any idea what they were doing[81]’

## Radiotherapy

- A. Francos: ‘I thought I would become radioactive ashes[82]’
- Valerie: ‘an incredible Star Wars piece of machinery[83]’
- Susan: ‘machines close to instruments of torture[84]’
- R. Thomason: ‘it’s worse than being shelled during the war[85]’
- E. Accad: ‘I have the feeling I am in a spaceship with scary nuclear weapons, the machine is making grilling noises[86]’; ‘it’s going to grill my skin[87]’
- F. Rubert: ‘an instrument of death[88]’
- Agent99: ‘my body and soul were just raped by treatment[89]’
- S. Tabet: ‘the dose might be too strong[90]‘. *In a dream*: ‘an iron machine that will swallow me[91]’. ‘black magic[92]’

The contents of these quotes suggest that overall, despite medical progress, the perceptions of the medical system and of the treatments it offers are extremely negative. The representations mentioned by those subjects can be divided into 6 categories:

---

[81] Norton, M. (2008). *Lopsided: How having breast cancer can be really distracting*. New York: Viking, p. 114.
[82] Francos A., ibid., p. 102.
[83] Kahane, D.H. *No less a woman: Femininity, sexuality, and breast cancer*. Alameda, CA: Hunter House Publishers, 1995, p. 34.
[84] Kuner S., Osborn C., Quigley L., Stroup K, ibid., p. 122.
[85] Thomason R., ibid., p. 296.
[86] Accad E., ibid., p. 193.
[87] Ibid., p. 221.
[88] Rubert F., ibid., p. 84.
[89] Pettason A., ibid., p. 140.
[90] Tabet S., ibid., p. 24.
[91] Ibid., p. 25.
[92] Ibid., p. 145.

- Fantasies of rape
- Violence, mutilation
- Representations of an enemy
- A poison
- Images of war such as bombings, torture, instruments of death, and Nazi camps
- Black magic, a demon, or a devil.

These testimonials suggest that the representations associated with the medical system, surgery, radiotherapy, and chemotherapy are intensely frightening. The therapeutic protocol and the medical context are viewed as threatening, violent, and sometimes even deadly. For instance, Joseph refers to a demonic torturer, Accad mentions scary nuclear weapons, and Tabet compares radiotherapy to a machine that will swallow her. Negative representations of the treatments also tellingly appear in some of the patients' dreams. Moreover, these representations are also explicitly associated with negative affect. For example, Francos mentions that she is terrified[93], Accad writes that the treatment 'is like being thrown over a cliff, she's terribly anxious[94]', Rubert feels like being 'in a slaughterhouse, she's very frightened[95], Tabet is petrified[96]. Thus, the negative perceptions of the medical system, of surgery, radiotherapy, and chemotherapy that can be found in those testimonials can have several harmful consequences on the patients' emotional states, quality of life, and disease outcome. The acute negative representations associated with the treatment protocol may result in pessimistic expectations and lasting negative affective states. Harboring such pessimistic representations can have a detrimental impact on adherence with treatment. Spiegel & Classen have observed that those perceptions can undermine confidence in medical interventions[97]. Indeed, various studies suggest that non-compliance to treatment is high among

---

[93] Francos A., ibid., p. 102.
[94] Accad E., ibid., p. 37.
[95] Rubert F., ibid., p. 46.
[96] Tabet S., ibid., p. 24.
[97] Spiegel L., Classen C. (2000). *Group therapy for cancer patients*. New York: Basic Books.

patients: Spiegel & Classen state that some cancer patients interrupt radiotherapy and chemotherapy treatment[98]. In one study, 23% of patients did not keep their appointments for the administration of chemotherapy. What's more, the withdrawal from the recommended treatment protocol is estimated to range from 16 to 23%. Therefore, it can be hypothesized that the lasting negative representations of treatments disclosed in autobiographies could have a detrimental impact on prognosis through frequent non-adherence to the treatment regimen. Moreover, these perceptions play an important role in the experience of the disease as they tend to impact behavior, affective states as well as the patient's immune system. as recent research in psychoneuroimmunology has shown. The ongoing negative experience generated by the representations of cancer treatments can lead to chronic tension, depression, anxiety, fear, and distress and therefore to the release of immunosuppressant catecholamines and a long-lasting imbalance between the sympathetic and parasympathetic systems. Negative feelings, such as fear, helplessness, despair, and rage can upset the endocrine balance, bring about over-activation of the hypothalamus-pituitary-adrenal axis, elevate the immunosuppressant hormone cortisol, and weaken the immune system.

## Perceptions of Lack of Support

In addition, numerous patients state that they feel unsupported, rejected, and sometimes even abandoned. Dakof & Taylor have observed that breast cancer patients often report rejection, withdrawal, and communication problems with their families and friends[99]. Indeed, according to Gelie, Barrault & De Castro, 43% do not feel understood by

---

[98] Ibid.

[99] Dakof, G. & Taylor, S. (1990). Victims' perception of social support: What is helpful for whom? *Journal of Personality and Social Psychology* 58 :1, 80-89.

their family, friends, and acquaintances[100], as we can see in the following quotes.

- Laura: "(my significant other) didn't know what to do: there were lots of emotional conflicts (…), he was not equipped emotionally, wasn't interested in trying to comfort me. I was very upset about that[101]", "He wanted the relationship over and terminated it. Disappeared. He didn't want anybody who had problems[102]"
- Sarah: "what I really needed was people who relieved me of the job of making them feel better, and who were able to listen both to my good and bad feelings[103]"
- Karen: "my fiancé became less and less hopeful about my recovery (…), he made plans that didn't include me (…) and became more reluctant to touch me. Our sexual relationship dried up. I thought I was physically repulsive. He stopped sitting on the couch next to me (…). Spending every day around someone who thought I was going to die soon made it difficult to believe otherwise[104]"
- C. Brunet: "I was looking for some support but I found a captain with an absent heart. Now the relationship is over[105]"
- Lilybelle2: "some people would give me the look like I was already given a death sentence and I could see the pity in their eyes. My sister-in-law, the one I'm closest to, would not even come to see me. She told me later that if she didn't see me, she wouldn't have to think of the cancer[106]"
- Mme jbc: "my real family was too busy, uninterested[107]"

---

[100] Gelie, F., Barrault, M. & De Castro, S. (2009). Rôle du coping, du soutien social général et spécifique sur la qualité de vie, l'anxiété et la dépression pendant les traitements pour un premier cancer du sein. In Cousson-Gelie, F., Langlois, E. & Barrault, M. (2009). *Faire face au cancer*. Paris: Tikinagan.

[101] Oktay, J.S. & Walter, C.A. (1991). *Breast cancer in the life cycle: Women's experiences*. New York: Springer, p. 85.

[102] Ibid., p. 87.

[103] Kahane DH., ibid., p. 9.

[104] Kuner S, Osborn C, Quigley L, & Stroup K., ibid., p. 136-7.

[105] Brunet C., ibid., p. 66-7.

[106] Pettason A., ibid., p. 230.

[107] Ibid., p. 68.

- Flower: "some very important people in my life such as family and friends have not wanted to share this journey with me. They have acted, from the beginning, as if I never had breast cancer[108]"
- Towanda2: "some of my close family members have been surprisingly distant[109]". "I'm very disappointed that (my mother) can't reach out to me and be supportive, she said: let's talk about something upbeat[110]"
- Doreen: "I lost my best friend, she didn't call (…) she couldn't handle the 'stress' of having a friend with cancer[111]"
- Lizzi: "my son: he'll change the subject (…), I feel lonely and separated from him when this happens[112]"
- Siggy001: "people I had always been around were no longer coming over or even calling. The turning point was when I was given a paper cup, plate and plastic silverware[113]"
- Janet: "my mother made the leap, got married, after my surgery in hospital, came to see me only twice! She basically began avoiding me[114]"
- Ro: "my significant other has been back pedaling as fast as he could to get out of the whole situation, adding to my depression[115]"
- Kathi1964: "my husband: dealing with his reaction to all of this would have been more devastating than the breast cancer itself[116]".

These quotes illustrate the trend towards perceived lack of social and emotional support (Sarah, Mmejbc, Kathi1964), isolation (Flower, Towanda2, Lizzi), rejection (Siggy001, Janet), and abandonment (Doreen, Laura, Karen, Brunet, Lillybelle, Ro) among western women who suffer from breast cancer. Seligman & Mason note that family members tend to

---

[108] Ibid.
[109] Ibid., p. 200.
[110] Ibid., p. 230.
[111] Ibid., p. 202.
[112] Ibid., p. 206.
[113] Ibid., p. 208.
[114] Ibid., p. 232.
[115] Ibid., p. 68.
[116] Ibid., p. 174.

distance themselves from the patient. In effect, Thierry states that only 10% of breast cancer patients benefit from an emotionally supportive network[117]. Research has shown that lack of social support and perceived loneliness have a nefarious influence on the individuals' quality of life and level of stress, which in turn can have a toxic influence on the person's mental health: for example, isolation and lack of social support are associated with higher rates of depression, longer depression and anxiety, reduced vitality and physical function. Perception of low social support is also related to high level of helplessness and distress. Moreover, Ozbay et al. have reported that social isolation is correlated with elevated heart rate and blood pressure, hypercortisolemia, and atherosclerosis[118]. Uchino, Cacioppo & Kiecolt-Glaser have noted that "the formation and disruption of social relationships have important immunological and endocrine sequelae in humans[119]", therefore poor social ties lead to negative medical outcome as isolation has a detrimental impact on the body's defense system. Conversely, Levy et al. note that higher NK activity is correlated with the perception of high-quality emotional support[120].

## General Consequences

More generally, from a physiological standpoint, ongoing negative affect such as feelings of isolation associated with the anxiety-provoking representations of breast cancer and its treatments disclosed in autobiographies may therefore indirectly influence not only mood and

---

[117] Thierry, A. (2005). *Les Effets des réseaux sur les représentations du cancer*, PhD., Sociology, University of Lille 1, France.

[118] Ozbay, F., Sharma, V., Kaufman; J., McEwen, B., Charney, D. & Soutwick, S. (2010). Neurobiological factors underlying psychosocial moderators of childhood stress and trauma. In R.A. Lanius, E. Vernetten & C. Pain dir. (2010). *The Impact of early life trauma on health and disease, the hidden epidemic*. Cambridge University Press.

[119] Uchino, B.N., Cacioppo, J.T. & Kiecolt-Glaser, J. (1996). The Relationship between social support and psychological processes: A review with emphasis on underlying mechanisms and implications for health. *Psychological Bulletin* 119: 3, 488-531.

[120] Levy, S.M., Herbermann, R.B., Whiteside, T., Sanzo, K., Lee, J. & Kirkwood, J. (1990). Perceived social support and tumor estrogen/progesterone receptor status as predictors of natural killer cell activity in breast cancer patients. *Psychosomatic Medicine* 52: 1, 73-85.

quality of life, but also outcome. Indeed, Corradi observes that the degree of stress experienced by the patient depends on the meaning of the illness[121], therefore we can hypothesize that the subjective perceptions of breast cancer, surgery, chemotherapy, and radiotherapy may lead to a robust nocebo effect. Indeed, Jaffe and Watkins have demonstrated that high levels of stress and negative emotional states have a neurochemical and neuroendocrine impact on the organism, resulting in the release of cancer-promoting chemicals such as pro-inflammatory cytokines, interleukin 6, catecholamines, and corticosteroids[122]. What's more, as research in psychoneuroimmunology has shown, the painful feelings resulting from intense negative representations and emotions can upset endocrine balance, elevate the immunosuppressant hormone cortisol and catecholamines[123] that play a crucial role in cancer cell destruction.

## PSYCHOTHERAPEUTIC INTERVENTIONS

Consequently, the current study explores the relevance of psychotherapeutic interventions to the negative emotions brought about by breast cancer as well as the subjective perceptions of the disease and its treatments. These aspects of the disease have implications for the use of psychological interventions designed for those patients. Currently, psychological support is often used by medical institutions in order to improve breast cancer patients' quality of life and coping skills as well as to reduce their negative affective states. I have attempted to clarify the potential practical applications of these interventions on the patients' representations of the disease and of the treatment protocol, as well as on their negative affect. According to Fawzy & Fawzy, a structured psychotherapeutic program consists of, among others, health education, stress management, training in active behavioral and cognitive coping, and

---

[121] Corradi, R.B. (1983). Psychological regression with illness. *Psychosomatics*, 24, 389-393.

[122] Watkins, A. (1997). *Mind-body medicine, a clinician's guide to psychoneuroimmunology*. New York: Churchill Livingstone.

[123] Borysenko, J. (1997). *Minding the body, mending the mind.* London: Bantam.

psychodynamic therapy[124]. First of all, psycho-education can provide face-to-face education about the disease, the symptoms, the treatment regimen, and its side effects[125]. Indeed, according to Petrie & Weinman, the first cause of problems related to radiotherapy and chemotherapy are due to insufficient preparation and information[126]: for example, in a sample of female patients given adjuvant radiation therapy, 23% did not know the name of the treatment. Therefore, psychoeducation can play a crucial role, as giving patients accurate, reassuring, and comprehensible explanations about breast cancer, such as the structure and the dynamics of cancer cells, the way treatments work, and the possible side effects, can lead to a more realistic view of the disease and thus reduce negative affect. The accurate information given by professionals also results in a better understanding of breast cancer therapies and alleviates the prolonged painful emotions that tend to be associated with the negative perceptions of the treatment. Thus, the implicit meaning attributed to the therapeutic protocol could be less negative. That in turn may contribute to more optimistic expectations, better quality of life, and more adequate coping. Psychoeducation can also deal with the mood disturbances caused by breast cancer, such as distress and anxiety[127]. In addition, these psychosocial interventions can promote a more positive outcome as their positive effects may enhance the body's disease-fighting and self-healing capacities through the psycho-neuro-immunological route. Indeed, Kaufman & Micha have noted that informed patients exhibit less fear, less distress, develop more effective coping strategies, and that their stress level is lower[128]. Paschali et al. have observed that the patients who were given information about the illness and the treatment reported more positive representations of the disease,

[124] Fawzy, I. & Fawzy J. (1995). A Short-term psycho-educational intervention for patients newly diagnosed with cancer. *Supportive Care for Cancer* 3, 225-228.

[125] Matsuda, A., Yamaoka, K., Tango, T., Matsuda, T. & Nishimoto, H. (2013). Effectiveness of psycho-educational support on quality of life in early-stage breast cancer patients: A systematic review and meta-analysis of randomized controlled trials. *Quality of Life Research*, 23, 21-30.

[126] Petrie K.J., Weinman J.A. *Perceptions of Health and Illness.* Amsterdam, Netherlands: Hardwood Academic Publishers, 1997.

[127] Matsuda, A., Yamaoka, Tango, Matsuda, & Nishimoto, ibid.

[128] Kaufman, E. & Micha, V.G (1987). A Model of psychotherapy with the good prognosis cancer patient. *Psychosomatics*, 28(10): 5340-548.

which led to improved physical and psychological functioning and better adaptation[129]. According to Spiegel & Classen, numerous studies have shown that a better access to information about the illness and the treatment protocol is also beneficial to the patients' compliance and therefore to the evolution of the disease[130].

What's more, psychotherapeutic interventions such as cognitive behavioral therapy and psychodynamic therapy can also contribute to the modification of the patients' maladaptive disease representations, which could become less emotionally burdening. Capozzo, Martinis, Pelis & Giraldi demonstrated that psychotherapy reduces anxious preoccupation[131] while Matsuda, Yamaoka, Tango, Matsuda & Nishimoto state that psychotherapeutic support improves emotional well-being and may bring about self-restorative reappraisal among breast cancer patients[132]. Moreover, Antoni notes that cognitive behavioral therapy is associated with lower cortisol levels and enhanced immune function[133]. In effect, numerous studies suggest that psychotherapy has robust health benefits: Burton & Watson point out that "social support is an important predictor of health in its own right[134]". Indeed, Pert writes that "when a sick person senses the care of another human being, their physiology changes: blood flow increases, heartbeat slows, breathing is enhanced, resulting in a healing state[135]". Interestingly, Moorey & Greer have observed that "long-term (cancer) survivors were found to have closer relationships[136]". For instance, married people tend to live longer and to develop better coping

---

[129] Paschali, A.A., Hadjulis, M. Papadimitrou, A. & Karade, E.C. (2015). Patient and physician reports of the information provided about illness and treatment: What matters for adaptation to breast cancer during treatment? *Psycho-oncology* 24: 8, 901-909.

[130] Spiegel, L., Classen, C. (2000). *Group therapy for cancer patients*. New York: Basic Books.

[131] Capozzo, M.A., Martinis, E., Pelis, G. & Giraldi, T. (2010). An Early structured psycho-educational intervention in patients with breast cancer: Results from a feasibility study. *Cancer Nursing* 33:3, 228-234.

[132] Matsuda, A., Yamaoka, K., Tango, T., Matsuda, T. & Nishimoto, H., ibid.

[133] Antoni M. (2013). Psychosocial intervention effects on adaptation, disease course, and bio-behavioral processes in cancer. *Brain, Behavior, and Immunity*, 30 (suppl.), 2013: S88-S98.

[134] Burton M. & Watson M. (1998). *Counseling people with cancer*. Chichester: Wiley, p. 29.

[135] Pert C. (2007). *Everything you need to know to feel good*. Carlsbad, CA: Hayhouse Publishers, p. 212.

[136] Moorey S. & Greer S. (1989). *Psychological therapy for patients with cancer: A new approach*. Oxford: Heinemann, p. 44.

skills. First of all, supportive connections favor positive health behaviors and greater compliance to treatment protocol. In addition, supportive relationships are generally associated with lower levels of stress, distress, hopelessness, anxiety, and depression, enhanced well-being, and fewer sleep disturbances.

Among the positive effects of psychotherapeutic interventions, Antoni also mentions that CBT techniques such as relaxation and stress-reduction practice are correlated with a 45% reduction in recurrence. Green Mc Donald, O'Connell & Lutgendorf have also established that the reduction of depressive symptoms achieved by CBT interventions confers survival benefits[137]. According to Uchino, there is a significant correlation between emotional support and lower cancer mortality[138]. In this respect, it is important to note that psychotherapeutic interventions can decrease the stress associated with the breast patient's perceived loneliness, distress, and anxiety, and enhance positive affective states and life satisfaction and thus provide a health-protective support. Therefore, developing psychotherapeutic interventions that include a high level of social support and empathy may have a beneficial effect on the patients' health status. Reduced stress due to the positive emotional state induced by the support provided by psychotherapeutic sessions also activates the left prefrontal cortex, which is associated with improved resilience and immune activity[139], greater natural killer cell cytotoxicity[140], and therefore enhanced self-healing abilities. In addition, positive mood decreases the level of inflammatory markers such as interleukin 6 and enhances natural killer cell cytotoxicity[141]. Thus, thanks to a reduction in negative mood, psycho-

---

[137] Green Mc Donald P., O'Connell M. & Lutgendorf S. (2013). Psychoneuroimmunology: A decade of discovery, paradigm shifts, and methodological innovations. *Brain, Behavior and Immunity* 30 March, 1-9.

[138] Uchino, B.N., Cacioppo, J.T. & Kiecolt-Glaser, J. (1996). The Relationship between social support and psychological processes: A review with emphasis on underlying mechanisms and implications for health. *Psychological Bulletin* 119: 3, 488-531.

[139] Antoni M., ibid.

[140] Michael YL, Berkman L, Colditz GA & Holmes MD. (2002). Social networks and health-related quality of life in breast cancer survivors: A prospective study. *Journal of Psychosomatic Research* 52: 5, 2002: 285-293.

[141] Pressman S, & Cohen S. (2005). Does positive affect influence health? *Psychological Bulletin* 133:6, 2005: 925-971.

educational, psychodynamic and cognitive behavioural interventions may also indirectly enhance immune function by improving natural killer cell activity. This aspect is particularly important since - as Doidge has pointed out - cancer is partly due to a failure of immune surveillance, which is modulated by neuropeptides responsible for the communication between the brain and the immune system[142]. Thus, maintaining a high level of immune competence is crucial for positive prognosis[143]. Supportive relationships also give rise to higher oxytocin production, which inhibits hypothalamic-pituitary-adrenal axis reactivity to stress. This in turn brings about lower cortisol levels, diminished epinephrine and norepinephrine release, and reduced sympathetic (fight-or-flight) reactivity. Ozbay et al. also point out that social support is an important resilience factor that may moderate the possible harmful impact of the social environment on gene expression[144]. Indeed, according to Kiecolt-Glaser & Glaser, McGuire & Robles, fear, distress, and depression can also bring about poorer repair of damaged DNA, increase the frequency of sister chromatic exchange, and result in alterations in apoptosis and poorer surveillance of abnormal cells[145].

## CONCLUSION

The negative perceptions of breast cancer and its treatments are an important aspect of the psychological experience of the disease. Although the results of the current study cannot be generalized due to small sample size, the selected breast cancer autobiographies show that for a significant number of patients, the illness is associated with intensely threatening and frightening representations. Moreover, these patients experience intense and lasting negative affect such as feelings of isolation, powerlessness,

---

[142] Doidge N. *The Brain that changes itself*. New York: Penguin, 2007.
[143] Watkins A., ibid.
[144] Ozbay et al., ibid.
[145] Kiecolt-Glaser J, Glaser R., McGuire L., Robles T.F. (2002). Psychoneuroimmunology: Psychological influences on immune function and health. *Journal of Consulting and Clinical Psychology* 70(3), pp. 537-547.

depression, and anxiety. This can have a detrimental effect on the patients' emotional balance, quality of life, and immune function. Therefore, this aspect of the illness should be given more attention and consideration by health care professionals. By creating a more realistic view of breast cancer, psycho-education, cognitive behavioral therapy, and psychodynamic psychotherapy can play a prominent role, because of its potential to provide emotional support, to reduce distress, anxiety, and stress and to improve coping skills and compliance to treatment protocol. Moreover, reducing the stress related to negative emotions and promoting more positive affective states can boost immune function and enhance the body's disease-fighting and self-healing abilities. Therefore, psychotherapeutic support that focuses on extensive information about the nature, evolution, and treatment of the disease, and on the enhancement of positive mood could be more widely used in medical institutions. Psycho-education about the disease as well as the treatment's goal and functioning could be generalized in order to give rise to more positive perceptions of the breast cancer therapies. Patients could be given access to individual psychotherapy in order to achieve better emotional support. This could have a beneficial effect on the patients' quality of life, compliance, adaptation, and disease outcome. Future research could explore the various modalities of psychotherapy used with breast cancer patients in order to determine the most efficacious types of interventions.

## REFERENCES

Accad, E. (2001). *The Wounded breast.* Melbourne: Spinifex.

Anagnostopoulos, F. & Spanea, E. (2005). Assessing illness representations of breast cancer: A comparison of patients with healthy and benign controls. *Journal of Psychosomatic Research*, 58, 4, 327-334

Andersen, B. L., Karlson, J. A., Anderson, B. & Tewfik, H. H. (1984). Anxiety and cancer treatment: Response to stressful radiotherapy. *Health Psychology*, 3, 535-551.

Anderson Copeland, C. (2000). *Coming through the darkness*. Springfield, MA: Destiny Press.

Antoni, M. (2013). Psychosocial intervention effects on adaptation, disease course, and bio-behavioral processes in cancer. *Brain, Behavior, and Immunity*, 30 (suppl.), 2013, S88-S98.

Ashley, L., Marti, J., Jones, H., Velikova, G. & Wright, P. (2015). Illness perceptions within 6 months of cancer diagnosis are an independent prospective predictor of health-related quality of life 15 months post-diagnosis. *Psycho-oncology*, 24, 11, 1463-1470.

Baker, G. K. (2008). *Cancer is a bitch*. Da Capo Lifelong Books.

Borysenko, J. (1997). *Minding the body, mending the mind.* London: Bantam.

Brunet, C. (2005). *La Vie vaut mille maux*. Quebec, Boucherville: Editions de la Mortagne.

Burton, M. & Watson, M. (1998). *Counseling people with cancer*. Chichester: Wiley.

Capozzo, M. A., Martinis, E., Pelis, G. & Giraldi, T. (2010). An Early structured psycho-educational intervention in patients with breast cancer: Results from a feasibility study. *Cancer Nursing*, 33, 3, 228-234.

Coquatrix, P. (1986). *Duel pour la vie*. Paris: Carrère Lafont. [*Duel for life*]

Corradi, R. B. (1983). Psychological regression with illness. *Psychosomatics* 24, 389-393.

Dakof, G. & Taylor, S. (1990). Victims' perception of social support: What is helpful for whom? *Journal of Personality and Social Psychology*, 58, 1, 80-89

De La Brosse, S. (1979). *La Force de vaincre*. Paris: Lattès. [*The Force to Overcome*]

Doidge, N. (2007). *The Brain that changes itself*. New York, NY: Penguin.

Fawzy, I. & Fawzy, J. (1995). A Short-term psycho-educational intervention for patients newly diagnosed with cancer. *Supportive Care for Cancer*, 3, 225-228.

Francos, A. (1983). *Sauve-toi, Lola.* Paris: Editions Bernard Barrault. [*Save yourself, Lola.*]

Freiman-Gibb, L. A., Janz, N. K., Katapodt, M. C., Zikmund-Fisher, B. J. & Northouse, L. (2016). Illness representations, risk perception, and fear of cancer recurrence in breast cancer survivors. *Psycho-oncology* 26, 9.

Gelie, F., Barrault, M. & De Castro, S. (2009). Rôle du coping et du soutien social général et spécifique sur la qualité de vie, l'anxiété et la dépression pendant les traitements pour un premier cancer du sein. In Cousson-Gelie, F., Langlois, E. & Barrault, M. (2009). *Faire face au cancer*. Paris: Tikinagan. [Role of coping and general and specific social support on quality of life, anxiety and depression during treatment for first-time breast cancer. In Cousson-Gelie, F., Langlois, E. & Barrault, M. (2009). *Coping with cancer*]

Green Mc Donald, P., O'Connell, M. & Lutgendorf, S. (2013). Psychoneuroimmunology: A decade of discovery, paradigm shifts, and methodological innovations. *Brain, Behavior and Immunity*, 30 March, 1-9.

Ireland, K. (2004). *Learning to trust myself, lessons from cancer and other dilemmas*. San Francisco: Wise Words Publications.

Jaffe, D. (1980). *La Guérison est en soi*. Paris: Laffont. [*Healing is in itself*]

Joseph, B. (1996). *My Healing from breast cancer.* New Canaan, Connecticut: Heats Publishing.

Kahane, D. H. (1995). *No less a woman: Femininity, sexuality, and breast cancer*. Alameda, CA: Hunter House Publishers.

Kaufman, E. & Micha, V. G (1987). A Model of psychotherapy with the good prognosis cancer patient. *Psychosomatics* 28(10), 5340-5348.

Kiecolt-Glaser, J., Glaser, R., McGuire, L. & Robles, T. F. (2002). Psychoneuroimmunology: Psychological influences on immune function and health. *Journal of Consulting and Clinical Psychology*, 70(3), pp. 537-547.

Knobf, M. T. (1986). Physical and psychologic distress associated with adjuvant chemotherapy in women with breast cancer. *Journal of Clinical Oncology* 4, 678-684.

Kuner, S., Osborn, C., Quigley, L. & Stroup, K. (1999). *Speak the language of healing: Living with breast cancer without going to war.* Berkeley, CA: Conari Press.

Linn, M. W., Linn, B. S. & Stein, S. R. (1982). Beliefs about causes of cancer in cancer patients. *Social Science and Medicine*, 16(7), 835-839.

Maillard Chaulin, B. (1999). *Journal d'un sein*. Orléans: Editions Corsaire. [*Diary of a breast*]

Matsuda, A., Yamaoka, K., Tango, T., Matsuda, T. & Nishimoto, H. (2013). Effectiveness of psycho-educational support on quality of life in early-stage breast cancer patients: A systematic review and meta-analysis of randomized controlled trials. *Quality of Life Research* 23, 21-30.

Mc Corry, N. K., Dempster, M., Quinn, J., Hogg, A., Newell, J., Moore, M., Kelly, S. & Kirk, S. J. (2013). Illness perception clusters at diagnosis predict psychological distress among women with breast cancer at 6 months post diagnosis. *Psycho-oncology* 22, 3, 692-698.

Michael, Y. L., Berkman, L., Colditz, G. A. & Holmes, M. D. (2002). Social networks and health-related quality of life in breast cancer survivors: A prospective study. *Journal of Psychosomatic Research* 52, 5, 285-293.

Moorey, S. & Greer, S. (1989). *Psychological therapy for patients with cancer: A new approach.* Oxford, UK: Heinemann.

Nethery, S. (1978). *One year and counting: Breast cancer, my world, and me*. Ada, MI: Baker Book House.

Levy, S. M., Herbermann, R. B., Whiteside, T., Sanzo, K., Lee, J. & Kirkwood, J. (1990). Perceived social support and tumor estrogen/progesterone receptor status as predictors of natural killer cell activity in breast cancer patients. *Psychosomatic Medicine* 52, 1, 73-85.

Norton, M. (2008). *Lopsided: How having breast cancer can be really distracting*. New York: Viking.

Ozbay, F., Sharma, V., Kaufman, J., McEwen, B., Charney, D. & Soutwick, S. (2010). Neurobiological factors underlying psychosocial moderators of childhood stress and trauma. In R.A. Lanius, E. Vernetten & C. Pain. (2010) dir. *The Impact of early life trauma on health and disease, the hidden epidemic*. Cambridge University Press.

Pachali, A. A., Hadjulis, M. Papadimitriou, A. & Karade, E. C. (2015). Patient and physician reports of the information provided about illness and treatment: What matters for adaptation to breast cancer during treatment? *Psycho-oncology* 24, 8, 901-909.

Pert, C. (2007). *Everything you need to know to feel good.* Carlsbad, CA: Hay House Publishers.

Pettason A. *I am not my breast cancer*. New York, NY: Harper, 2008.

Pressman, S. & Cohen, S. (2005). Does positive affect influence health? *Psychological Bulletin* 133, 6, 925-971.

Prevost, F. (1975). *Ma Vie en plus.* Paris: Stock. [*My Life in addition*.]

Rozema, H., Vollink, T. & Lechner, L. (2009). The Role of illness representations in coping and health of patients treated for breast cancer. *Psycho-oncology* 18, 8, 849-857.

Spiegel, L. & Classen, C. (2000). *Group therapy for cancer patients*. New York: Basic Books.

Rubert, F. (2006). *La Vie est là, simplement*. Paris: Albin Michel. [*Life is there, simply*]

Russell Rich, K. R. (1999). *The Red devil: To hell with cancer*. New York: Crown Publishers.

Sarton, M. A. (1997). *Recovering*. London: Women's Press.

Seligman, L. & Mason, G. (1996). *Promoting a fighting spirit: Psychotherapy for cancer patient survivors and their families*. Upper Saddle River, NJ: Prentice Hall Editors.

Shook, R. L. (1983). *Survivors: Living with cancer*. New York: Harper and Row.

Spiegel, L. & Classen, C. (2000). *Group therapy for cancer patients*. New York: Basic Books.

Tabet, S. (2010). *Les Patientes*. Paris: Les Empêcheurs de penser en rond. [*The patients*]

Thierry, A. (2005). *Les Effets des réseaux sur les représentations du cancer*, PhD., Sociology, University of Lille 1, France. [*Effects of networks on representations of cancer*]

Thomason, R. (2000). *Shoring up my soul: A year with cancer*. West Conshohocken, PA: Infinity Publishing.

Uchino, B. N., Cacioppo, J. T. & Kiecolt-Glaser, J. (1996). The Relationship between social support and psychological processes: A review with emphasis on underlying mechanisms and implications for health. *Psychological Bulletin* 119, 3, 488-531.

Vaillant, M. (2008). *Une Année singulière avec mon cancer du sein*. Paris: Albin Michel. [*A special year with my breast cancer*]

Watkins, A. (1997). *Mind-body medicine, a clinician's guide to psychoneuroimmunology*. New York: Churchill Livingstone.

In: Psychotherapy
Editor: Hayley Boyd

ISBN: 978-1-53618-877-6


*Chapter 8*

# ADOLESCENT PSYCHOTHERAPY AND CONVERSATION ANALYSIS

***Lautaro B. Barriga**, PhD***
Escuela de Psicología,
Universidad Bernardo OHiggins,
Santiago, Chile

## ABSTRACT

Psychotherapy has been shown to be an effective treatment that contributes to individual change and well-being; however, information on how therapeutic change is occurring in depressive adolescents is scarce. Recent studies of psychotherapy show that the study of the process from the therapeutic interaction provides clues to know the subjective dynamism of the patients by focusing on the conversation of the interlocutors. In this sense, the chapter shows a Structure of Therapeutic Conversational Exchanges that allows us to know the internal organization of the dialogues of successful psychotherapies of depressive adolescents with suicide attempts in a hospital context, segmenting the sessions in three main phases and analyzing the time occupied in the

* Corresponding Author's E-mail: laupsi@gmail.com.

production of intra and inter-process exchanges. The exchanges present different movements during the sessions and different moments when they are applied, which are related to the usefulness within the psychotherapy process. This knowledge allows the psychotherapist to know which, when, how to use and manage the Conversational Therapeutic Exchange Structure.

# 1. Introduction

## 1.1. Psychotherapy: From the Result to the Process

In the first half of the $20^{th}$ century, Eysenck questioned the effectiveness of psychotherapy, which prompted a significant and systematic increase in research focused on therapeutic effects and outcomes, proving that people who received treatment from a psychologist showed significant clinical improvement (Krause, Aristegui & De la Parra, 2002). During the second half of the 20th century, the efficacy of psychotherapy was confirmed when compared to placebos treatments and the absence of treatment, that is, it was demonstrated that its effect is significantly superior to the spontaneous remission of the symptom and those who receive psychological support improve in comparison to those who do not receive it. In this sense, the World Health Organization (WHO) recognizes psychotherapy as an effective treatment that promotes well-being and health (WHO, 2013). However, new questions arise that seek to link psychological models with the strength of therapeutic change, that is, it is attempted to know which of them is the most effective. The studies in this line brought up the paradox of equivalence or lack of differentiation, that is, it is shown that the different models or psychotherapeutic approaches produce a similar or homogeneous effect (Krause, 2005). What is interesting is that this paradox drives the:

a. Development of novel methodologies that increase knowledge and therefore a greater understanding of the effects of psychotherapy;
b. Development of evidence-based research in psychotherapy and;

c. In-depth exploration of the psychotherapeutic process (Krause, Aristegui, De la Parra & Strasser, 2006).

These methodological and investigative developments in psychotherapy allowed the introduction and approach to the comprehensive and interpretative analysis of the construction of meaning, that is, the studies of psychotherapy begin to be oriented towards the search of how the helping relationship is produced, assembled and functioning, which begins to be understood as a process centered on the therapeutic interaction that will allow for answering questions related to the therapeutic change and opening the possibility of realization:

a. Research that focuses on the changes presented by the patient and that are related to concepts that belong to a specific school of psychotherapy;
b. Research that focuses on the changes presented by the patient and that cannot be typecast in the theories of a specific school of psychotherapy, since they transcend and cross the different therapeutic concepts (Ress et al, 2001; Krause & Dagnino, 2005).

The study of the therapeutic process can be understood and addressed by approaching the patient's experience, the psychotherapist's experience, and the coordination of experiences of both interlocutors.

## 1.2. The Psychotherapeutic Process

In the last two decades, process studies have been concerned with understanding change in psychotherapy and for this purpose they focus on the moments and micro-moments that appear as significant and relevant in therapeutic interaction, with the aim of understanding in detail the strategies, interventions and actions that the psychotherapist carries out to coordinate with the patient and thus acquire knowledge about the alliance, dialogues, relationships, obstacles and facilitators of subjective change at the verbal and non-verbal levels (Krause & Dagnino, 2005). The objectives of process studies are:

a. Identify therapeutic episodes or events of progression and stagnation
b. To set off alarms about the existence of a conflict, difficulty, problem, suffering or traumatic experience;
c. Recognize in the difficulty, problem or traumatic experience the type of interventions or actions used by the psychotherapist;
d. Recognize the direct or indirect actions of the patient in responding to the psychotherapist's intervention;
e. Identify results during the course of the session that can be interpreted according to the theory on which the intervention is based (Poch & Avila, 1998; Krause, 2005).

Consequently, in order to carry out research on the psychotherapeutic process, it is necessary to identify the relevant segments or episodes that deliver signals of effective interventions, in order to decode them and make them intelligible to understand the therapeutic change. In the search for this understanding, methods of analysis must be considered that allow us to go beyond the classic methodology, as Cornejo (2005) suggests. Comprehensive and interpretative methods must be incorporated to account for the verbal and non-verbal language that is activated in the different therapeutic interventions.

Verbal language has been widely studied and presents different ways of understanding it, one of which is the view that goes beyond formal logic and that in the 1960s began to be developed under the name of Giro pragmático del lenguaje (Echeverría, 2006).

The pragmatic turn as a theoretical development focuses on the importance of the use and meaning of language in social interactions and has had a great impact on the world of psychology, especially psychotherapy, coming to establish the relationship: language and change (Jimenez, 2012).

The theory of the turn of language sees the human being as a linguistic being, who inhabits, lives, self-constructs, self-generates and invents himself alone and from language, to the point of becoming the key to understanding the different phenomena of human interaction (Echeverría, 2006). In addition, the turn of language allows us to understand that the human being is a hermeneutic being, that he understands and interprets himself by situating his existence in a specific space of the world (Arciero, 2009), in this way, language assumes the role of re-configurator with the property of altering the course of historical-social situations, Emerging the meaning of the lived and giving the possibility that the diachronic experience can be brought to the word or who speaks is the one who is experiencing, and in this sense the spoken and dialogued becomes the main focus of psychotherapy that needs to be studied by innovative methods such as Conversation Analysis (Jimenez, 2012; Villalta, 2009).

## 1.3. Conversation Analysis

The process of psychotherapy can be addressed by the "Conversation Analysis" (CA) initiated by Harvey Sacks and Emanuel Schegloff in the 1960s at the University of California, Berkeley. The CA is a comprehensive model that allows to approach, focus and deepen the analysis of verbal and non-verbal language of the situations experienced, facilitating the recognition of the different actions that allow the construction, coordination and articulation of the dialogues that are assembled in the continuous movement of the different moments and micro-moments of human interactions. The authors structure the AC method by studying the interactive behaviors of people who communicated by phone to the Suicide Prevention Center belonging to a University, observing that in each inter-communication that people made when they called, they did so to refer to and understand themselves and others, realizing that in each interaction the different ways of understanding the rights, duties and obligations of the different actors who are located in the same intersubjective space are tried to be manifested by means of verbal and non-verbal emissions that are linked to each other and organized in particular sequences in the different segments that make up speech (Sack, Schegloff & Jefferson, 1974: Peräkyla, 2004). These observations made it possible to demonstrate that the behaviors of people in formal and informal everyday situations are reasonable and can be decoded by procedures that are intelligible by methods shared by the interlocutors during the interaction and that are useful insofar as they make it possible to communicate, to confirm one's own identity, to recognize one's own behavior and that of others (Pomerantz & Fehr, 2000; Peräkyla, 2011). In each interaction, the behavior of the interlocutors is aligned to the immediate and specific contingencies of the moment. In this sense, the contribution of each interlocutor allows the construction of a continuous understanding that emerges from the interactive actions and that in turn determines the future behavior of the interlocutors, since they will recognize ways of decoding verbal and non-verbal emissions that are linked in the intersubjective space and that give way to particular interactive sequences that are mutually comprehensive within the segments of speech, and that the authors called it: "Interaction Structure of the Adjacent Pair or the Basic Sequence" (Sack, Schegloff & Jefferson, 1974: Peräkyla, 2004). The Adjacent Pair is a basic organization of two speech actions, where the first action of one speaker invites a particular and specific type of second speech action to be performed by the other speaker, mobilizing and generating the dialogue that is interwoven with non-verbal expressions, Thus, for example, we can find that before a question there is a possible answer, to an invitation a possible acceptance, among others, putting in an explicit way the way of understanding the rights and the duties of the people when entering in contact, and this way of mutual understanding is a way of operating that is presented successively (Gaete, Aristegui & Krause, 2017). In this sense, the CA acquires the property of being a model of analysis that offers the possibility of investigating both verbal and non-verbal or paralinguistic interaction, such as phrases, sentences, sound quality, pauses, silences, turns, new beginnings, postures, movements, facial expressions, among others, as it enters the micro-moments of different situations, as for example in the psychotherapeutic encounter, the researcher can access and stop in the specific segments to investigate and deepen the process, with the purpose of understanding the organization and structure of the dialogues that facilitate the emergence of meaning and the change that takes place during the therapeutic conversation in different patients and especially with adolescents (Peräkyla, 2004; Gaete, Aristegui & Krause, 2017).

## 1.4. Adolescent Psychotherapy and Mental Health

With respect to adolescent psychotherapy, it should be pointed out that studies of processes are still scarce in this age group, finding some conceptual descriptions such as the therapeutic alliance, emotional well-being, the figure of the psychotherapist, specific skills and others that are based on studies of adult patients, demonstrating the need to study the process of therapeutic change in adolescents (Vargas, Gumucio & González, 2015; Cortés, Fernández, Capella & Krause, 2018). Consequently, interventions with adolescents must be based on evidence with specific therapeutic strategies that incorporate the characteristics and needs of this evolutionary period, since it is a particular and complex stage that is marked by physical, psychological and social changes that are oriented towards reaching socio-emotional maturity (Páramo, 2011; Parra, 2005). These changes impact individual, family, sexual, school and social functioning, challenging the psychological organization of the adolescent, which must deploy various adaptive and homeostatic processes to articulate the disturbances and contribute to the generation of healthy growth and development. However, for different situations the adaptation mechanisms are not sufficient to maintain the balance of the individual system, generating the risk of an unprotective and unhealthy adolescent process that leads to the installation of discomfort, discomfort and mental illness (Paramo, 2011; Vicente et al, 2012).

With respect to mental illness, adolescents in recent decades have shown a significant increase in prevalence. Global statistics show that 20% of adolescents suffer from mental health problems, that depression is the clinical picture that most contributes to the burden of disease among young people, and that suicide is the second leading cause of death among 10-29 year olds in the general population, and the third leading cause of death in adolescent males (Silva, 2019; Guajardo, Ojeda, Achui & Larraguibel, 2015).

Chile's statistics indicate that we are the second country in the world and the first in Latin America that has increased its suicide rates the most. Suicide ideation is present in up to 62% of young people, with the documentation that of every three adolescents in secondary school who think that life has no meaning, two of them think about committing suicide and one of them tries it, which reflects the strength of this phenomenon that has increased steadily between 1993 and 2012 in ages ranging from 10 to 19, going from 6 to 12 cases of suicide for every 100. This is the third leading cause of death among adolescents after accidents and homicide (Organization for Economic Cooperation and Development [OECD], 2013; Guajardo, Ojeda, Achui & Larraguibel, 2015). These figures indicate the importance of this phenomenon in the adolescent population, worrying numbers that have led the Ministry of Health of Chile (MINSAL) to consider it a public health problem and that through its National Health Strategy for the decade 2010 to 2020 has incorporated adolescent suicide as a health objective, in order to reduce its rates through actions that allow early detection of cases at risk, improve the quality of care, train health personnel and sustain assistance in crisis situations (MINSAL, 2014). The emphasis of the MINSAL is on prevention, on the importance of health care and the therapeutic approach by the mental health services belonging to the public and private network at their different levels of care (primary, secondary, tertiary), establishing that according to the severity of the suicide attempt which can be mild, moderate, serious and extreme, the tertiary health system or hospital assistance will be the device in charge of responding to adolescent suicide attempts from the serious and extreme indicator (MINSAL, 2013).

Inpatient adolescent mental health services, depending on the severity of the suicide attempt, offer outpatient and inpatient care to adolescents with suicide attempts. It is worth mentioning that in both services the main indication is psychological intervention (Almonte, Correa & Montt, 2012; Guajardo, Ojeda, Achur & Larraguibel, 2015).

According to the background presented, the questions that have guided Barriga's investigations (2019) have been: How is the psychotherapeutic conversation of adolescents with depressive disorders and suicide attempts organized? How is the therapeutic change armed and structured in successful processes of change?

# 2. The Research

## 2.1. Psychotherapy, Conversation Analysis and Exchange

As mentioned, the CA facilitates the study of the psychotherapeutic process, since a- Conversation, when considered as an action, allows the visibility of the movements and transfers of all the elements of human activity, such as emotions, intentions and words that are produced in the interactive encounter of the interlocutors; b- This action is organized, that is, the interlocutors in the activities of social life are organized from the dialogue to reach the objectives and; c- Conversation maintains Intersubjectivity, that is, the physical space is transformed into a relational space that promotes the coordination between the interlocutors so that they reach their purposes (Peräkyla, 2004). These ideas have allowed psychotherapy researches to use the AC analysis method to understand the therapeutic conversation that has been organized from a linguistic unit called "Conversational Exchange."

To talk about the Exchange it is necessary to mention one of the main representatives of the interactional linguistics Catherine Kerbrat-Orecchioni (1998), who points out a- The components of the interaction that facilitate the understanding of the interlocutors are the communicative framework and the rules of the conversation; b- The notion of interaction allows the development of the ideas of the Conversational Exchange and the mutual influence of the interlocutors, where talking is exchanging and exchanging is talking and; c- The structure of the verbal interaction groups five elements of the conversation, which in turn form two communicational units or hierarchical structures that are

a. Dialogical units or the dialogical dimension of language that involves different interlocutors who are in the same interactive space in which the dialogue is constituted. This dimension includes the phases of interaction, the thematic sequences and the exchange. It is necessary to have a minimum of two interlocutors interacting.
b. Mono-logical units that correspond to the contribution made by each interlocutor who is participating in the dialogue. This dimension includes the interventions and the speech acts. It is necessary to have at least one interlocutor. (Kerbrat-Orecchioni, 1998; Villalta, 2009)

A study carried out by Barriga (2017) considers the Conversational Exchange as the unit of interactive language that links the dialogical dimension with the mono-galgal dimension. In this sense, the Exchange constitutes an interactive bridge that is capable of reflecting how the interlocutors reach shared meanings, building cooperative actions, organize their contributions in dialogues and obtain interactive satisfaction in the process of psychotherapy, in addition to being dependent on the context in which they are produced and presenting temporal delimitation according to specific themes, they are configured as the central axis of the conversation whose knowledge is relevant to advance in the strategies of psychotherapists and to walk towards therapeutic change. From this point of view, the investigations that are detailed show the internal organization of the therapeutic conversation and how the change is armed and structured from the unit of the Conversational Exchange in complete psychotherapeutic processes of depressive adolescent women with a suicide attempt considered to be of high severity and who received attention in a hospital setting.

## 2.2. Method

### *2.2.1. Research Design*

We used the qualitative method with an exploratory and descriptive design inserted in the line of the interactive linguistics, combining techniques of qualitative ethnographic cut with quantitative elements that are associated to observation records of complete psychotherapy processes.

### *2.2.2. The Participants*

Multiple case study with intentional search for participants who fit the study objectives. The cases corresponded to two complete psychotherapy processes that were carried out in a child and adolescent mental health service of a public hospital, and were made up of the following participants:

- *Case 1:* Formed by: a) Clinical Psychologist with studies in Social Constructionism, certified by the National Commission of Clinical Psychologists, with 10 years of seniority in the hospital mental health service and more than 13 years of experience in the care of children and adolescents and; b) Adolescent female, 15 years old, 2 months of age, in secondary education, with a diagnosis of severe depression according to the International Classification of Diseases in its tenth version (ICD-10), admitted to the hospital for presenting severe suicide attempts.
- *Case 2:* Formed by: a) Clinical Psychologist with studies in the Integrative approach, certified by the National Commission of Clinical Psychologists, with 10 years of seniority in the hospital mental health service and more than 8 years of experience in the care of children and adolescents and; b) Adolescent female, 15 years old, 6 months of age, attending secondary school, living with a responsible adult and with a diagnosis of severe depression according to the ICD-10, derived from the emergency service for making a serious suicide attempt.

### *2.2.3. Unit of Analysis*

Of the categories of conversation analysis, the Conversational Exchange was used as the unit of analysis, which corresponds to the binding unit of the interactive dimensions of language in interaction. A psychotherapeutic investigation of Barriga (2017) with adolescents with depressive disorders in a hospital setting allowed the creation of a "Structure of Therapeutic Conversational Exchanges" that organized the dialogues produced in the psychotherapy process and which were grouped into six types of Exchanges that were validated and graphed with examples (Table 1). Each session was divided internally into phases or time sequences called beginning, development and closing, in which the Exchanges were analyzed.

### *2.2.4. Information Processing*

Two complete psychotherapy processes were worked on, and from a total of twenty-eight sessions, sixteen were analyzed, eight for each process and selected in the following way: the two sessions at the beginning, four sessions of the development and the last two sessions, thus guaranteeing the representativeness of the case studies. The sessions were filmed in audio-video with two cameras in fixed and synchronized mode at the time of analysis, one directed at the psychologist and the other at the adolescent. Since the interaction between psychologist and patient is highly dynamic, a procedure of continuous observation of the Exchange Structure categories was chosen, therefore time stamps were made every 5 seconds during the course of the sessions. By using this procedure, it was possible to analyze the associations, frequency, duration, proportion and differences in the real time occupied in the production of each category of the Exchange Structure that was recognized in the segmentation of the sessions from an intra and inter-process psychotherapy perspective. For the decoding of the collected data, the Videograph computer software was used (Rimmele, 2009) that allowed the organization of the information in the same unit. The analysis of the inter-observer agreement was carried out with the Kappa index, obtaining 0.842 (good) for the Exchange Structure Categories and 0.823 (good) for the Phases that segmented each session.

To analyze the significance of the associations, the non-parametric statistical tools of Pearson's Chi-square (X2) were used, which were complemented with Cramer's V coefficient to diminish the bias of the sample sensitivity. In social sciences, values above 0.30 indicate moderate significant association (Manzano-Arrondo, 2017). The data was also analyzed from the dependence of the cases with statistical significance between the categories by means of the corrected typed residue and the differences of the typed variables. In this sense, the relationship level of the categories was determined as $Z = \pm 1.96$. The Mann-Whitney U test was used for the comparative analysis of the intra- and inter-process sessions.

### 2.5. Ethical Procedure

The protocols were adjusted to the requirements of the health studies and were approved for execution by the hospital's bioethics committee. The respective informed consents and assents were signed.

## 3. Results

The results are presented around the "Structure of Therapeutic Conversational Exchanges," which allowed to analyze the busy times and the mutually dependent movements that took place in the different sessions that were located in a hospital context. The analysis was made on a total of 5,396 units of exchanges recognized in the time segments counted in both psychotherapy processes. Each session was divided into three major phases of time that were called: a- Beginning which corresponds to the first moments of the meeting, in general they are spaces in which adherence is strengthened and doubts about the session are resolved; b- Development which corresponds to the interventions and psychotherapeutic work that will be responsible for leading to change and; c- Closing where the psychologists give signals that the session is ending, reflect the relevance of the topics discussed, prepare the farewell and invite to a next session. It is worth mentioning that the beginning and closing phases are temporarily brief and both phases are characterized by inviting therapeutic work and by sustaining the bonding, whereas the developmental phase is temporarily extensive and in it the psychotherapeutic work is carried out. The production of the Exchanges in the different phases presents variations in the occupation of time, observing that in the phase of development there is greater production of the Subjective Story Exchange in both psychotherapy processes, reaching approximately a third of the total production of the Exchanges counted (34.4% and 30.2% respectively). Also noteworthy is the Adherence Exchange, which appears with a constant production in both psychotherapy processes and with greater concentration in the beginning and closing phases (79.5% and 64.2% respectively) (See Table 2).

A statistically significant relationship was found between the "Structure of Conversational Therapeutic Exchanges" and the phases that segmented the sessions of the psychotherapy processes [Chi-square (4,N = 5,396) = 76,39; $p < 0.001$], with a moderate dependency force (V of Cramer = 0.301). From this it can be inferred that there is an interdependence between the Exchange Structure and the phases of each psychotherapy session. It is observed that the distribution of time of the Exchange Structure with the phases of initiation, development and closure are statistically different (U of Mann-Whitney = 317,733,55.141; $p < 0.001$), which indicates that the occupation of time in the production of Exchanges in the different phases in both processes are sensitive to this Structure. In addition, significant differences are appreciated in the times destined to the production of Exchanges between psychotherapy processes ($Z = 2.56$; $p < 0.05$). The corrected typed residues of the boxes of the Exchange Structure show that the Exchanges of Symptom Exploration, Subjective Telling, Context Exploration and Self-Knowledge are independent of the phases of beginning and closing of the sessions in both therapeutic processes. It is worth mentioning that the analysis of the percentages in the boxes shows that the beginning and closing of the sessions concentrate a greater amount of time in the Adherence Exchange, while in the development phase a greater amount of time is invested in the Subjective Story and Self-Knowledge Exchange as shown in Table 2.

**Table 1. Structure of Therapeutic Conversational Exchanges**

| N | Exchanges | Definition |
|---|---|---|
| 1 | Adherence. | They are dialogues that promote bonds, sometimes they are extra-therapeutic and transmit warmth, confidence and comfort.<br>Example:<br>1. Psychotherapist 1: .............You know you are very close (smile).<br>2. Patient 1: (pause) Really<br>3 .Psychotherapist 1: Of course, (pause) You are very talented and you will get through this (smile).<br>4. Patient 1: I hope, I think I can with your help, thank you very much. (Patient 1, extract from Adhesion Exchange, start phase, 00:01:35 - 00:02:40) |
| 2 | Exploration of the symptom | They are dialogues to obtain information about the history of the symptom, its development and behavior.<br>Example:<br>1. Psychotherapist 2: Ahh, (pause), at some point you told me that you cut yourself and became intoxicated ........<br>2. Patient 2: Yes, (pause) eeehh, I want to (pause) die<br>3. Psychotherapist 2: yaa. (pause)When did you start with this?<br>4. Patient 2: A couple of years ago,<br>5. Psychotherapist 2: (silence), eehhh, (pause)......(Patient 2, extract from Symptom Exploration Exchange, developmental phase, 00:13:15 - 00:15:02). |
| 3 | Subjective story. | They are dialogues that invite to narrate the experiences. Example:<br>1. Psychotherapist 1: (Talking about the friend), (silence) What do you think about this?<br>2. Patient 1: I don't know, I think it wasn't right, I thought we were friends... and nothing, I was wrong.<br>3. Psychotherapist 1: (silence) mm (pause). And something else......<br>4. Patient 1: ehhh, I remember that she always told me that we would be together, it was so nice when we went out in the summer to the square, always together....<br>5. Psychotherapist 1: (Silence), yaaaa...<br>6. Patient 1: I remember that that day in the square we met some kids and we told them things that were lies and they believed us, then they invited us to eat ice cream and drink, we enjoyed that day a lot.<br>7. Psychotherapist 1: It seems that way and what else do you remember...(Patient 1, extract from Interchange of subjective story, developmental phase, 00:25:16 - 00:27:07) |

**Table 1. (Continued)**

| N | Exchanges | Definition |
|---|---|---|
| 4 | Exploration of the context. | They are dialogues to obtain information from the patient's context such as: family, school, etc. Example:<br>1. Psychotherapist 2: (Talking about friends)...., Ok, (pause) and......<br>2. Patient 2: My friends are from the street.<br>3. Psychotherapist 2: How many?<br>4. Patient 2: I have several, all homeless, they're all torn out.<br>5. Psychotherapist 2: Ok<br>6. Patient 2: (Silence) but others I know online<br>7. Psychotherapist 2: (Silence) How old are they (pause)?<br>8. Patient 2:.........(Patient 2, excerpt from Context Exploration Exchange, developmental phase, 00:09:21- 00:12:15) |
| 5 | Self-knowledge | They are dialogues to deepen and articulate the patient's disturbing emotional experiences. Example:<br>1. Psychotherapist 1: (Talking about the problem with the friend) mmmm. (Silence) What happens to you when you talk to me about this?<br>2. Patient 1: (Silence). I don't know, it's strange......(pause)<br>3. Psychotherapist 1: (Silence). Mmmmm. How strange, how so?<br>4. Patient 1: (Silence) Eeeeee, mmmmmm, I don't know, these are things that are difficult for me to describe, (pause), Eeeee.... I don't know how to explain it, (pause), it's something that overwhelms me (pause)<br>2. Psychotherapist 1: (pause), How does that invade you (Patient 1, self-knowledge exchange extract, developmental phase, 00:19:02 - 00:22:19) |
| 6 | Explanation of the other's problem. | These are dialogues to agree and agree on the patient's internal states such as: discomfort, suffering, confusion, etc. Example:<br>1. Psychotherapist 2: (talking about the family). I think that when you try to resolve your .....you confuse.<br>2. Patient 2: (Silence). Can be (pause) yes<br>3. Psychotherapist 2: (Silence). Look, every time we talk and you've told me about problem situations, I've seen you try to solve them, but something happens that you can't solve (pause), you seem to block yourself,<br>4. Patient 2: (Silence). Yes, you are right, I block, (pause) and react badly (Patient 2, excerpt from Exchange of explanation of the problem of the other, development phase, 00:21:07 - 00:23:00). |

Adapted from: Barriga, L. 2017.

## Table 2. Time of exchanges by session segmentation of psychotherapy processes 1 and 2

| Structure of Exchange | Start | Process 1 Development | Close | Total 1 | Start | Process 2 Development | Close | Total 2 |
|---|---|---|---|---|---|---|---|---|
| 1- Adherence. | 79.5[5. 6] | 8.4[3.7] | 64.2[2.8] | 18.3 | 70.4[-5.6] | 5.3[-3.7] | 54.3[-2.8] | 12.2 |
| 2- Exploration of the symptom | 0.5[-0.7] | 9.8[-2.1] | 8.1[-0.9] | 8.5 | 0.2[0.7] | 18.4[2.1] | 16.3[0.9] | 16.4 |
| 3- Subjective story. | 1.2[-1.2] | 41.1[-7.2] | 9.4[-1.9] | 34.4 | 2.2[1.2] | 37.0[7.2] | 12.2[1.9] | 30.2 |
| 4- Exploration of the context | 18.4[3.3] | 11.1[1.6] | 6.2[-1.1] | 11.7 | 24.8[-3.3] | 19.4[-1.6] | 6.4[1.1] | 17.9 |
| 5-Auto-Knowledge | 0.2[0.6] | 19.2[6.4] | 1.2[0.6] | 15.8 | 0.6[-0.6] | 15.1[-6.4] | 0.3[-0.6] | 11.6 |
| 5- Explanation of the other's problem. | 0.2[-1.7] | 10.4[3.1] | 11.9[2.0] | 11.2 | 1.8[1.7] | 4.8[-3.1] | 10.1[-2.0] | 11.7 |
| Total % | 100 | 100 | 100 | 100 | 100 | 100 | 100 | 100 |

Adapted from: Barriga, L & Villalta, M. 2019.

A statistically significant relationship is also observed between the psychotherapy processes and the Exchange Structure [Chi-square (5,N = 5,396) = 45,39; $p < 0.001$], with a moderate dependency force (Cramer's V = 0.333). This allows us to infer that the Exchange Structure is interdependent with psychotherapeutic processes located in a hospital context. The comparison of the distribution of the times used in the production of Exchanges with the psychotherapeutic processes is statistically different (U of Mann-Whitney = 24,555,667.544; $p < 0.001$). Therefore, it is inferred that each psychotherapist constructs and organizes the Exchanges in a different way, which affects the times that are occupied by Exchanges. Other statistically significant differences are observed in how the production of exchanges is distributed between sessions of the psychotherapy processes (U of Mann-Whitney = 25,478,125.557; $p < 0.005$).

Significant differences are observed in the times destined to produce Exchanges when comparing the 1st with the 5th session and then between the 9$^{th}$ and 14$^{th}$ session, either intra-process ($Z = 3.18$; $p < 0.01$) and between processes ($Z = 2.87$; $p < 0.04$), from which it can be inferred that the amount of exchanges is different between the compared sessions of the same process and also between the compared sessions of different therapeutic processes.

From the comparative analysis of the corrected typified residues of the boxes of the Structure of Exchanges of the 1st and 5th session separated by processes, it is inferred that in process 1 the Exchanges of Exploration of the symptom and Exploration of the context are independent of the psychotherapy processes, while in process 2 only the Exchange Exploration of the symptom is independent. Furthermore, in the 1st session of both processes, psychotherapists invest more time in the Adherence Exchange (19.1% and 15.7% respectively) and less time in the Self-Knowledge Exchange (0.5% and .01% respectively), while in the 5th session, in both processes more time is invested in the Self-Knowledge Exchange (29.2% and 22.6% respectively).

In addition, from the comparative analysis of the corrected typified residues of the boxes of the Exchange Structure of the 9th and 14th session, it is observed that the Symptom Exploration and Context Exploration Exchanges are independent in both psychotherapy processes and that the Self-Knowledge Exchange occupies less time in the last session in both processes (18.6% and 15.2% respectively). Finally, the percentages in the boxes indicate that the Adherence and Subjective Story Exchange present a stable production during the sessions analyzed in both processes.

## CONCLUSION

The research shown was focused on the time that the different Exchanges occupied in two complete processes of psychotherapy of adolescents with suicide attempts attended in a mental health service of the child and adolescent belonging to a hospital enclosure. The exchanges in terms of Kerbrat-Orecchioni (1998) constitute the minimum dialogical unit, which, by understanding it as a unit that links interlocutors who are mutually oriented, allows the configuration of dialogical structures. The research used the Structure of Therapeutic Conversational Exchanges that Barriga raised in a study of 2017 in a hospital context, and then proceeded to segment the sessions in three phases that are: beginning, development and closure to analyze the time spent in the production of exchanges during the interactive process that characterizes the cooperative action and thus obtain greater understanding of how the Structure of Exchanges moves during the psychotherapeutic conversation of depressed adolescents.

The exchanges were dealt with according to the usefulness that the psychotherapists perceive in developing their interventions, in this sense that one Exchange is more sensitive than another to the type of objective and intervention that is being carried out with the patients.

By occupying more time in the Adherence Exchange at the beginning and at the end of each session in both psychotherapeutic processes, it can be maintained that the well-being and comfort of the patient is a requirement that must be present in each session and that it is the psychotherapist who has to promote these dialogues to guarantee the support of the therapeutic alliance that is sustained in the mutual coordination and synchronization between the verbal contributions of each interlocutor and that also repairs the roughness that may have arisen in the therapeutic encounter. It is thought that the Adherence Exchange constitutes the best support for conversational meetings, and is an essential psychotherapeutic strategy that lays the foundation for building change. This is in accordance with the theories of Rogers (1969), Orlinsky & Howard (1986), who emphasize that psychotherapeutic success requires the development of a good alliance and therapeutic adherence.

It is striking that the Self-Knowledge Exchange is little occupied in the first and last session and that it is independent of the beginning and closing phases, but with a high occupation in the developmental phase, which allows us to infer that this Exchange is exclusive to psychotherapeutic work and that its production is conditioned by adherence, symptom exploration and context. Then, guaranteed the above, it is possible to access, mobilize and articulate different emotional content of the adolescent, which would explain its greater presence in the developmental phase and in intermediate sessions. This is coherent with Guidano (1999), who refers to the fact that the psychotherapist focuses and works in and with the emotional world of the other person to generate change and that emotional disturbances need time to work and articulate them. Therefore, the use of the Self-Knowledge Exchange is strategic, one must know at what moment to use it, since this type of Exchange works with the deepest subjective contents of the other, consequently the psychotherapist must be very conscious when opening and closing these dialogues. In this sense, its use is with caution and prudence.

The exchange of Subjective Storytelling presents the greatest occupation of time and a stable production during the processes of psychotherapy. Therefore, psychotherapists generate a dialogue that allows the adolescent to remember and progressively describe the contents of her life in order to obtain a wide and precise knowledge of the experience of the other. In this sense, it seems that this Exchange is for the psychotherapist a transversal axis that provides, mobilizes and connects information that configures a general scenario of the adolescent. This is in agreement with Peräkyla (2004), who proposes that in the intersubjectivity of the conversation history is being constructed and understood.

It is important to emphasize that the Exchanges of Exploration of the symptom and Exploration of the context occupy more time in the 1st session and are independent of the process, which allows us to infer that they are useful mainly at the beginning of the psychotherapeutic process, perhaps because the symptoms and the context are superficial contents, easily accessible and recognized by the adolescents, therefore these dialogues help to lower the resistance and increase the fluidity of the conversation. Discussing topics that are easily recognized by the interlocutors favors the coordination of actions, and the different verbal emissions pave the way for addressing deep issues (Pomerantz & Fehr, 2000).

It is reasonable to think that there are differences found in the times of production of the Exchanges between processes, since psychotherapists when applying their theoretical models will present different forms in the contact, in the language and in the techniques, but that they do not affect the content of each exchange. Nevertheless, future studies should deepen the relationship between times of production of Exchanges and the psychotherapeutic school.

It can be stated that the Structure of Therapeutic Conversational Exchanges presents a permanent movement described in the therapeutic processes, but that they are adjusted to the work of the psychotherapist in the interaction with the interlocutor. The knowledge generated helps the clinician to consider that: a) There are more functional Exchanges at the beginning of the process, such as the Exploration of the Symptom and Exploration of Context. b) There are Exchanges that should be promoted throughout the process, such as Adherence. c) There are Exchanges that are used with caution in addressing the emotional world, such as Self-Knowledge. d) This knowledge allows the psychotherapist to know what, when, and how to use this Structure.

Finally, it is important to continue developing and seeking greater precision of the "Structure of Therapeutic Conversational Exchanges" that was described, and to investigate other dialogical structures that may account for other disorders with different age groups and psychosocial conditions.

## REFERENCES

Almonte, C. and Montt, M. E. (2012). *Child and adolescent psychopathology (2nd edition).* Ed. Mediterráneo, Santiago.

Arciero, G. (2009). *Selfhood, Identity and Personality Styles.* Editorial. Wiley.

Barriga, L. (2017). The Change in Psychotherapy: Analysis of the Conversation in Psychotherapies with female adolescents hospitalized for attempted suicide in a hospital in the Metropolitan Region of Chile. *(Thesis for the degree of Doctor of Psychology),* Doctoral Program, School of Psychology, University of Santiago de Chile.

Barriga, L. and Villalta, M. (2019). Conversation Analysis: Psychotherapy of depressive adolescents with suicide attempts in a hospital setting. *Psychological Therapy*, 2019; 37(1), 39-51.

Barriga, L. and Villalta, M. (2019). The psychotherapeutic conversation of novice and expert. An exploratory study in Chile. *Argentine Journal of Psychological Practice,* 2019; 28(V), 703-713.

Cornejo, C. (2005). The two cultures in psychology. *Journal of Psychology of the University of Chile*, 14(II):189-208.

Cortés, A., Fernández, O., Capella, C., Espinosa, H. and Krause, M. (2018). What Changes in Psychotherapy? The Perspective of Adolescent Patients with Depressive Symptoms, Their Therapists and Outdoor Observers. *Psykhe, 27*(II): 1-15.

Echeverría, R. (2006). *Ontology of language. Santiago*: JC Sáez editor.

Gaete, J., Aristegui, R. and Krause, M. (2017). Four conversational practices to promote a change of therapeutic focus. *Revista Argentina de Clínica Psicológica*, 28(II): 220-231.

Guajardo, N., Ojeda, F., Achui, L. and Larraguibel, M. (2015). Therapeutic Interventions for Suicidal Behavior in Adolescents1. *Rev. Chil. Psiquiatr. Neurol. Infanc. Adolesc*, 26(II): 145-155.

Jiménez, A. (2012). *The effectiveness of the word on interpretation and the processes of subjective change in psychotherapy.* Thesis for the professional title of Psychologist. University of Chile.

Guidano, V. (1999). *Development of Post-Rationalist Cognitive Therapy. Santiago: Institute of Cognitive Therapy.*

Kerbrat-Orecchioni, C. (1998). *Verbal interactions. Interactional approach and structure of conversations. Volume I. (Third Edition).* Armand Colin. Paris, France.

Krause, M., Aristegui, R., & De la Parra, G. (2002). *Towards an effective practice in Psychotherapy: study of relevant episodes of change in different types of psychotherapy and their effects on therapeutic outcomes FONDECYT Project.* Santiago: School of Psychology, Pontificia Universidad Católica de Chile.

Krause, M. (2005). *Psychotherapy and change, a look from subjectivity.* Santiago de Chile: Ediciones Universidad Católica de Chile, 2005.

Krause, M. & Dagnino, P. (2005). Evolution of change in the psychotherapeutic process. In R. Riquelme & E. Thumala (Eds.), *Advances in Psychotherapy and Psychic Change* (pp. 21-35). Santiago, Chile: Chilean Society of Mental Health.

Krause, M., Aristegui, R., De la Parra, G. and Strasser, K. (2006). *Acilitating change in psychotherapy: effective and ineffective communicational interactions in different psychotherapeutic modalities.* Project funded by FONDECYT Nº 1060768.

Manzano-Arrondo, V. (2017). *Chi cuadrado de Pearson para dos variables nominales.* Recuperado de http://asignatura.us.es/dadpsico/ apuntes/ChiCuadrado.pdf.

Ministerio de Salud de Chile (2013). *National Suicide Prevention Program: guidelines for its implementation Department of Mental Health,* Division of Disease Prevention and Control, Under Secretary of Public Health.

Ministerio de Salud. Government of Chile. Deis/minsal (2014). *Available at: http://deis.minsal.cl. National Health Strategy for the fulfillment of the Health Objectives of the Decade 2011-2020 (MINSAL).* Available at: http://web. minsal.cl/portal/url/item/c4034eddbc96c a6de0400101640159b8. Pdf. 2015.

Organización Mundial de la Salud (2013). *Mental health: a state of well-being.* Retrieved from http://www.who.int/features/factfiles/mental_health/es/index.htm.

Organization for Economic Cooperation and Development (OCDE) (2013). *Health at a Glance. OECD Indicators.*

Orlinsky, D., & Howard, K. (1986). Process and outcome in psychotherapy. En: S. Garfield y A. Bergin (Eds.), *Handbook of psychotherapy and behavior change* (3ra. Ed.). New York: Wiley.

Páramo, M. (2011). *Risk factors and protective factors in adolescents*: Content analysis through discussion groups Electronic version]. *Revista Terapia Psicológica*, 29,(I): 85-95.

Parra, A. (2005). *Family and adolescent development: a longitudinal study on evolutionary trajectories*. Thesis for the PhD in Psychology, University of Seville.

Peräkyla, A. (2004). Two traditions of interaction. Department of Sociology, University of Helsinki, Finland British. *Journal of Social Psychology* 43: 1–20.

Peräkyla, A. (2011). After interpretation: Third position utterances in psychoanalysis. *Research on Language and Social Interaction*, 44 (III): 288-316.

Poch, J., & Ávila, A. (1998). *Research in psychotherapy. The psychoanalytic contribution.* Barcelona: Paidós.

Rees, A., Hardy, G. E., Barkham, M., Elliott, R., Smith, J. A. and Reynolds, S. (2001). 'It's like catching a desire before it flies away': A comprehensive process analysis of a problem clarification event in cognitive-behavioral therapy for depression. *Psychotherapy Research,* 11:331-351. doi:10.1093/ptr/11.3.331.

Rogers, R. (1957). The necessary and sufficient conditions of therapeutic personality change, *Journal of Consulting Psychology*, 21: 95-103.

Rimmele, R. (2016). *The program for coding of videos.* Recuperado desde www.dervideograph.de.

Sack, H., Schegloff, E., & Jefferson G. (1974). A simple's systematics for the organization of turn-taking for conversation. *Language,* 50(IV): 696-735.

Silva, L. (2019). Child and adolescent suicide: a warning for the fulfillment of the global imperative *Acta Paulista de Enfermagem*, *32*(III), III-IVI.

United Nations Children's Fund [UNICEF], (2012). *Fourth study of child abuse. Santiago: UNICEF.*

Vargas, B., Gumucio, F., & González, C. (2015). Effectiveness in therapeutic interventions with children and adolescents Factors associated with the Person of the Therapist and the Therapeutic Alliance. *Rev. Chil. Psiquiatr. Neurol. Infanc. Adolesc*, 26(II): 7-10.

Vicente, B., Saldivia, S., De la Barra, F., Melipillán, R., Valdivia, M., & Kohn. R. (2012). Child and Adolescent Mental Health in Chile and Health Care Gaps. *Rev Med Chile*; 140, 447-57.

Villalta, M. (2009). Conversation Analysis. A proposal for the study of didactic interaction in the classroom. *Journal of Pedagogical Studiess,* 35(I): 221-238.

In: Psychotherapy
Editor: Hayley Boyd
ISBN: 978-1-53618-877-6


*Chapter 9*

# PSYCHOTHERAPY FOR MOTHERS AND THEIR CHILDREN: LESSONS LEARNED FROM THE EFFECTIVENESS STUDIES

***Cansu Alsancak-Akbulut****
Department of Psychology, Ankara University, Ankara, Turkey

## ABSTRACT

Motherhood is a challenging life phase for any woman. Mothers' need for support for childbearing and the risk of psychological disorders increase during this life phase. It is well-known that mothers with mental illnesses usually do not provide sensitive and affectionate parenting to their infants and children (Frigerio et al., 2019). Thereby, children and families may also experience critical negative consequences. For instance, previous studies consistently demonstrated that marital satisfaction is lower among depressed mothers and their husbands (Barnes, 2006). Furthermore, maternal depression is associated with children's insecure attachment and negative representations of self (Teti et al., 1995; Toth et al., 2009). These negative consequences may intensify when the mothers' psychological disorder goes untreated.

* Corresponding Author's E-mail: cakbulut@ankara.edu.tr.

Therefore, intervening with these mothers and providing them effective treatment have critical importance for them and their families. Previous literature has displayed various forms of intervention and psychotherapy programs for mothers and their children. These programs included group-based and individual-based psychotherapy for decreasing the level of maternal depression and increasing psychological well-being (e.g., Grote et al., 2008; James, 2002; Kersting et al., 2003; Swartz et al., 2016). Furthermore, several intervention programs were conducted with depressed mothers to promote secure attachment and developmental competence in children (e.g., Cicchetti et al., 1999; 2000). In light of the literature, this chapter aims to review the effectiveness and efficacy of these psychotherapy and intervention programs conducted with mothers and their children. This chapter will inform families to seek effective treatments and researchers to advance their intervention methods and techniques, which contribute to the healthy development of society.

**Keywords:** mothers, children, effectiveness, psychotherapy, intervention

## INTRODUCTION

Parenting is one of the major roles and developmental tasks of individuals (Luster and Okagaki, 1993), therefore parenthood is likely to be one of the main sources of one's sense of self (Stern, 1995). Birth giving provides mothers with the responsibility to raise a child, who behaves in accordance with the rules of society and becomes a functional member of the community. Since several psychosocial and physiologic changes occur during perinatal and postnatal periods in women, it seems plausible that caregiving would be challenging and stressful for nearly all mothers. A sizeable number of mother experiences parenting stress and/or psychological disorders during pregnancy and/or child-rearing. Parents tend to have substantially higher rates of depression either before or after childbirth relative to national norms. Unfortunately, less than half of the parents with clinically depressive symptoms receive mental health services (Gopalan et al., 2010). In addition to depression, the rates of anxiety are also likely to increase during the early years of child-rearing (Romans-Clarkson et al., 1988). Especially, being a single mother (Kotwal &

Prabhakar, 2009), and having lower levels of socioeconomic status (Brown & Moran, 1997; Kotwal & Prabhakar, 2009) seem to increase the risk for the likelihood of psychopathology.

Depression during pregnancy (Field et al., 2000; Koutra et al., 2013) and maternal psychopathology, in general, are associated with an increased risk of psychopathology in children, such as internalizing and externalizing behaviors (Mesman et al., 2017), as well as their negative developmental outcomes (e.g., emotion dysregulation, lower levels of self-esteem, aggression, a decline in intelligence, negative interpersonal relations; Cicchetti & Toth, 1995; 1998). Mothers having higher levels of psychopathology symptoms are also likely to be emotionally unavailable and have a nonsynchronous relationship with their children (Licata et al., 2016). Furthermore, maternal depression is associated with children's insecure attachment and negative representations of self (Teti et al., 1995; Toth et al., 2009). In addition to negative developmental and relationship outcomes, maternal psychopathology is closely linked to decreases in marital satisfaction (Barnes, 2006). Given the impact of maternal psychopathology on developmental child outcomes, mother-child relationship, and marital quality; these outcomes are more likely to become chronic if these mothers do not obtain any psychological and/or psychiatric treatment. Previous research has demonstrated that greater attention should be paid to translating existing knowledge on developmental and clinical theories in designing and applying preventive and treatment-focused interventions so that these might remediate the detrimental effects of maternal/child psychopathology and ineffective parenting practices on children. Therefore, the present chapter aims to review the effectiveness of mother-child psychotherapy and intervention programs and address the lessons learned from these studies.

Various psychotherapy and intervention efforts, which are specifically applied to mothers or mother-child dyads, have been developed and implemented over the past few decades. Historically, Mahler (1973) and Winnicott (1971) were the pioneers of developing treatment programs to rehabilitate infants and mothers simultaneously. Fraiberg (1980) also applied a systematic treatment to mother-infant dyads and proved to the beneficial effects of examining mothers' parenting practices, and using infants as catalyzers of therapeutic changes (as cited in Cramer, 1995). All these efforts lead to elaboration on the approaches and conceptualizations of mother-child psychotherapy and interventions. Nowadays, various therapeutic and intervention models, which focus on the mothers (Grote et al., 2008), children (Blake, 2018), and mother-infant dyads simultaneously (Fonagy et al., 2016), have been applied. Furthermore, various therapeutic methods and techniques have been developed to fulfill the psychological needs of mothers and their children. Grounded on all these theoretical background, this chapter presents the types of mother-child psychotherapy and intervention, as well as recent studies showing the effectiveness of these approaches. Specifically, this chapter includes attachment-based interventions, individual and group psychotherapy approaches, and psychoeducation programs. Finally, the lessons learned from all these studies are discussed for their potential contributions to the healthy development of mother-child dyads and society.

## Psychological Treatment Approaches for Mothers and Their Children

### Individual Psychotherapy

Individual psychotherapy sessions with mothers and/or their children have been applied extensively to decrease the level of psychopathology symptoms and increase the psychological well-being of families. Individual psychotherapy usually targets mothers with psychological disorders, mothers of children with psychopathology, and children having adaptation problems. All these services designed specifically for parents were named as "psychotherapy of parenthood" by Sutton and Hughes (2000). According to these researchers (Sutton & Hughes, 2005), there are two purposes of psychotherapy of parenthood: (1) assisting parents during childbearing years so that they can develop effective parenting approaches and improve the relationship with their child, (2) fulfilling the needs of the child that the parents cannot fulfill effectively. In addition to these purposes, it can be argued that decreasing the level of parental psychopathology to decrease its spill-over effect on the parent-child relationship and child psychopathology may be another essential purpose of the psychotherapy efforts.

The salutary effects of psychotherapy with parents, especially with mothers, have been reported by several effectiveness studies and case reports (Grote et al., 2008; Gruber et al., 2006). For instance, a meta-analysis, including eight trials, most of which include mothers with postpartum depression, demonstrated the favorable effect of psychological treatments for maternal depression (effect size = 0.35; Cuijpers et al., 2015). Another study focused on mothers of school-aged children and showed that interpersonal psychotherapy is effective in decreasing maternal mood symptoms and impairment in children as compared to mothers treated in treatment as usual (Swartz et al., 2008). Previous studies also showed decreases in internalizing and externalizing behaviors of children having parents with mental disorders as a result of preventive interventions (see Siegenthaler et al., 2012 for a meta-analysis). For instance, Swartz et al. (2016) applied two different forms of brief psychotherapy (brief interpersonal psychotherapy and brief supportive psychotherapy) to the mothers with depressive symptoms and found that there is a link between improvement in mothers' depressive symptoms and their children's functioning. The results of these studies indicate that individual psychotherapy for mothers with psychological disorders is an effective treatment for alleviating psychopathology symptoms of mothers and in turn, their children.

In their study, Cooper and Murray (1997) randomly assigned mothers into four conditions, which are cognitive-behavioral therapy, dynamic psychotherapy, non-directive counseling, and routine primary care. Except for routine primary care, all groups reported improvement in maternal mood and decrement in relationship difficulties at the end of the interventions. However, this study demonstrated that mother-child face-to-face engagement and attachment security could not be enhanced in any of these groups. Similarly, Fonagy et al. (2016) conducted a randomized controlled trial of psychoanalytic psychotherapy for parents with mental health problems and their infants. They found no differences over time between groups on maternal reflective functioning, parent-infant interaction, and infant development. However, they proved that psychoanalytic parent-infant psychotherapy was effective in improving maternal mental health and decreasing parenting stress. These findings indicate that psychotherapy for parent-child dyads might be effective in enhancing the well-being of parents and improving mental health, however this effect does not appear to translate into promoting the positive parent-child relationship.

## Group Psychotherapy

The evidence to date indicates that higher levels of social support help to increase life satisfaction and decrease relationship problems of mothers and their children with psychological disorders (Abel et al., 2005; Marsack & Samuel, 2017). These findings may support that group psychotherapy, in which a group of individuals participates in the group process in the manner to obtain favorable therapeutic gains, would be beneficial for parents. The group psychotherapy process may help parents to experience therapeutic growth thanks to the therapeutic alliance between the group members and therapist. Therapeutic alliance within the group involves compatibility, support, caring, trust, and mutual liking, all of which are likely to produce favorable therapeutic outcomes (Burlingame et al., 2001). In addition to a group supportive experience, group psychotherapy has various advantages. For instance, group psychotherapy is usually less costly and there are less attrition rates.

Armstrong et al. (2003) described the Parents for Youth group treatment approach for parents of adolescents with disruptive behavior disorders. The group included a maximum of twelve parents, who meet a weekly basis for one and a half hours. This group treatment was designed for assisting the parents to gain awareness about the discrepancies between them and their youth rather than to "control" or "change" them. It was argued that during the safe, supportive, empathic, and non-blaming group process, parents gained insight into the factors that intensify the relationship difficulties with their children and enhanced their sense of hope while lessened shame, fear, anger, and guilt. Thereby, by emphasizing gaining control of themselves rather than their children, Parents for Youth served as a protective factor to reduce disruptive behavior disorders. Similarly, Gruber et al. (2006) conducted group psychotherapy combining psychoeducational, supportive, and psychodynamic approaches with parents of patients with schizophrenia. In line with the findings of Armstrong et al. (2003), they found that reliving high levels of anger, fear, and sorrow in parents and re-establishing their socioemotional balance help to reduce problems at home. This group process suggests that creating a supportive, empathic, and non-blaming atmosphere is beneficial for parents to gain awareness of their inner processes with their children and use this insight in their interactions with their children. A supportive group process provides mothers with a favorable environment, in which they can freely observe their inner thoughts and feelings.

Group psychotherapy may be used as an "add on" treatment to the standard psychiatric treatment for mothers with psychological disorders. Luthar and Suchman (2000) examined the effectiveness of the relational psychotherapy mothers' group, which was designed to serve heroin-addicted mothers. Relational psychotherapy mothers' group, which combined developmental psychoeducation and supportive psychotherapy, was carried out additionally to standard methadone counseling. This approach aimed at promoting optimal parenting by addressing mothers' psychosocial vulnerabilities. This add on treatment was found to be effective in decreasing the risk for child maltreatment and increasing maternal involvement and positive psychosocial adjustment over time. This study demonstrates that a group psychotherapy approach can be incorporated into a standard psychiatric treatment of at-risk mothers. In another study, Field et al. (2000) suggested that providing childcare for vulnerable mothers may improve their relational problems with their children. In their study, while infants of Afro-Caribbean and Hispanic adolescent mothers with depression received all-day care, mothers participated in intensive social/vocational rehabilitation program. This approach was found to be associated with the better mood in mothers and better mother-infant interactions. A similar approach, which aimed to integrate psychiatric treatment into the daily routine of mothers with neurotic disorders, was conducted by Kesting et al. (2003). While mothers received psychoanalytical-interactional group therapy, art therapy, body therapy, and consultation on weekdays, their children were cared for by a child-care worker. The results showed that there is an improvement in the mothers' symptom levels, everyday functioning, and psychosocial problems. Although the generalizability of these findings is questionable, these approaches may indicate that providing mothers with multiple effective treatments, which fulfill their current psychological and social needs, can improve their relational difficulties. Furthermore, integration of group therapy to standard treatments may be a favorable substitute to inpatient treatment, which has several disadvantages for mothers with infants and children.

## Attachment-Based Parenting Interventions

In recent years the attempts to develop and implement attachment-based intervention programs to enhance the healthy mother-child relationship and remediate maternal or child psychopathology have been increasing (Dozier & Roben, 2015; Juffer et al., 2017a; 2017b). These intervention programs are grounded on the premise that the early childhood period is essential in forming the capacity to be securely attached to the main caregiver(s). Early interactions and experiences with the caregiver provide children with opportunities to explore the environment and be protected when they are distressed (Bowlby, 1969/1982). Mothers, who recognize and understand their child's signals and respond to them in appropriate and prompt manner (i.e., be sensitive), are more likely to have securely-attached children (Ainsworth et al., 1978). Grounded on the attachment theory, the overarching goal of these intervention programs is to promote positive interactions among mother-child dyads to ameliorate the emergence of child psychopathology (Ialongo et al., 2006).

Various attachment-based interventions are proved to be effective in enhancing the interactional quality of mother-child dyads through video-based techniques, which aid mothers through modeling and observation. Video-based interventions include various forms, such as Video Microanalytical Therapy, Video Interaction Guide, and Video-feedback Intervention to Promote Positive Parenting (Juffer et al., 2008; Hynd & Kahn, 2006; Tilley & Chambers, 2000), and are applied to mothers with various psychopathology, including depression (Hynd & Kahn, 2006) and bulimia nervosa (Stein et al., 2006). Mothers are treated using different approaches within the parenting interventions, including behavioral approach and representational approach. The behavioral approach focuses on modeling and providing video-feedback to mothers to promote positive parenting (Knoche et al., 2012; van IJzendoorn et al., 1995). Whereas, in the representational approach interveners address the mother's attachment experiences with their own parents or maternal representations on the mother-child relationship (Baradon et al., 2005; Frost, 2012). Nowadays, various attachment-based interventions use either behavioral or representational approach while providing mothers with psychoeducational materials, or intervene at both levels.

Several meta-analytic reviews investigated the effectiveness of attachment-based programs, which were applied to many vulnerable groups (Bakermans-Kranenburg et al., 2003; 2005; Fukkink, 2008). Bakermans-Kranenburg et al. (2003) concluded that the methods that include behavioral sensitivity, shorter duration (less than 6 sessions), and video-feedback are more effective than the representational approach, longer durations, and interventions without video-feedback. However, previous literature involves randomized controlled trails that contradict the effectiveness of using behavioral approach alone. For instance, Cicchetti et al. (2006) conducted a randomized controlled trial of psychodynamic mother-infant psychotherapy and found that the representational approach is effective in increasing attachment security and reducing attachment disorganization. Indeed, it should be noted that although the meta-analysis of Bakermans-Kranenburg et al. (2003) found that the behavioral approach is more effective than the representational approach, this meta-analysis included only one study focusing on the representational approach. In addition, given that maternal representations may change in longer time periods as compared to behaviors, the effectiveness of the representational approaches may be hard to detect statistically. A psychotherapy program targeting infants with feeding programs and their mothers showed its effectiveness only at a 6-month follow-up. Wan et al. (2008) reported that representational approaches that aim to enhance mother-child interaction quality are effective in altering the attachment patterns of children, whereas discussing their attachment state of minds with mothers does not seem to be effective. Therefore, using hybrid models that combine behavioral and representational approaches may result in the most effective outcomes.

There is some indication that one of the determinants of these interventions' effectiveness may be the problem areas that they are focusing on. For instance, Stein et al. (2006) applied a video-feedback interactional treatment to mothers with bulimia nervosa. They found improvements in the mother-child interactions during mealtime, however the intervention did not show effectiveness in ameliorating maternal psychopathology. Similarly, in their study focusing on Interaction Guidance Treatment, which was grounded on cognitive-behavioral therapy, Murray et al. (2003) proved that the treatment is effective in reducing the relational problems among mothers and their infant, but not in increasing maternal sensitivity. However, focusing especially on enhancing maternal sensitive behaviors, Video-Feedback Intervention to Promote Positive Parenting (VIPP) was found to be effective in increasing maternal sensitivity (Juffer et al., 2017a; 2017b). These findings may infer that attachment-based interventions can be effective in reducing maternal or child psychopathology through promoting positive parenting practices and child attachment security.

## Psychoeducational Interventions

Psychoeducational approach involves training mothers didactically in general child development, parenting skills, stress management strategies, and development of social support networks (Cicchetti et al., 2006). Bristol et al. (1993) examined the effect of a psychoeducational intervention on the depressive symptoms of mothers of children with autism spectrum disorders. The intervention program was designed to help mothers to gain insight on children's disorder and to learn how to deal with the children's problem behaviors. Modeling, reinforcement, and feedback were the main techniques that were used during the course of intervention. Results of this study showed that maternal depressive symptoms and child problem behaviors decreased over time in the intervention group as compared to the control group. Psychoeducational interventions to change parents' attitudes towards corporal punishment were also proved to be effective. Either applied via psychoeducational books or videos, these interventions demonstrated a significant decrease in mothers' corporal punishment attitudes (Reich et al., 2012; Scholer et al., 2010). For instance, Holland and Holden (2016) examined the efficacy of a psychoeducational program, which was grounded on motivational interviewing and applied in a one-time individual session. The aim of this program was to change the positive attitudes toward corporal punishment, behavior intentions, and actions (e.g., spanking, slapping to the child). The findings supported that only one session of the psychoeducational program is effective in decreasing positive attitudes and intentions toward corporal punishment. These studies supported the notion that psychoeducation programs may be effective in teaching mothers adaptive coping strategies when they have children with certain disabilities, and in changing their attitudes toward child-rearing approaches.

Other studies also demonstrated improvements in maternal and child outcomes as a result of psychoeducational efforts, however high-risk groups may be exceptions to this impact (Tessier et al., 1998). Smith et al. (2005) compared socially disadvantaged mothers, who were randomly assigned to intervention and information-only group to examine whether a responsive parenting intervention is associated with the preintervention parenting resources. Results showed that receiving developmental information and advice was not effective in improving responsiveness among mothers with higher levels of depression and hostility. In another study, Juffer et al. (2005) applied a video-feedback intervention to adoptive families to promote positive parenting in addition to providing them with a personal educational book. The results showed that the educational book did not reduce the disorganized attachment in infants as opposed to the sensitivity-based intervention. These studies may demonstrate that training at-risk mothers via educational resources or giving them advice are unlikely to translate into better relationship quality and attachment organization.

## CONCLUSION

This chapter aims to review the effectiveness and efficacy of psychotherapy and intervention programs targeting mothers and their children. Individual and group psychotherapy approaches, parenting interventions, and psychoeducational programs are presented within the scope of this chapter. These approaches to mother-child psychopathology and relationship difficulties use a variety of methods and techniques, which are designed to fulfill the treatment needs of mother-child dyads. Research seeking to identify and evaluate these approaches suggest that positive changes in maternal and child psychopathology and parent-child relationship quality are achievable, although there are numerous challenges of making observable changes in these areas in high-risk groups. Highlighting the implications of these psychotherapy and intervention efforts, this chapter informs families to seek effective treatments and researchers to advance their intervention methods and techniques, which contribute to the healthy development of society.

In developing and implementing psychotherapy and intervention approaches, mother-child dyads' emerging needs and characteristics, as well as etiological factors that may have contributed to their psychopathology must be considered. Specifically, while psychotherapy and interventions with the representational approach were shown to be effective in decreasing the level of psychopathology symptoms and parenting stress of mothers, interventions with the behavioral approach suggest more positive changes in maternal sensitivity and mother-child relationship quality. When maternal psychopathology or/are attachment insecurity become potential risk factors for ineffective parenting practices, long-term individual/group psychotherapy efforts and representational approaches may be more effective in alleviating the problems in the family. After earning success by using these approaches, clinical interventions may aim to improve positive parenting and relational outcomes by incorporating both the mother and child into the process. Since, previous meta-analyses consistently suggested that mother-child relationship quality and maternal sensitivity are more effectively increased with the implementation of behaviorally-focused short term parenting interventions (Bakermans-Kranenburg et al., 2005; Juffer et al., 2017a; 2017b), relational interventions for mothers and their children may be one of the best approaches to enhance positive parenting (Nylen et al., 2006). Furthermore, given the complexity of difficulties and characteristics of targets, a personalized approach, which tailors intervention methods and techniques in accordance with the emerging needs of mother-child dyads, may be essential.

The characteristics of targets of psychotherapy and intervention programs should be considered before implementing these approaches. Clinical approaches involving a high emotional or cognitive load may not be effective for mothers with a severe psychological disorder or living in poverty, since these mothers may have difficulties in maintaining the treatment programs or their symptom levels may increase. Thereby, there may be difficulties in achieving observable changes in mothers and children in high-risk groups. These groups may require additional support systems and resources for gaining the favorable outcomes of the clinical interventions. Additional treatments to the standard psychiatric treatments for families in at-risk groups may result in more effective outcomes compared to isolated or standard clinical interventions. For instance, providing children of mothers with highly distressed and exhausted all-day child care also help them refresh and relieve their stress while working on their inner processes with the help of clinicians or interveners. It should be noted that the additional approaches to the treatment should fulfill the current needs of the mothers. Evidence is limited for the effectiveness of providing educational resources in promoting positive outcomes in mother-child dyads in at-risk groups (Juffer et al., 2005; Smith et al., 2005), although educational programs found to be effective in changing mothers' attitudes and teaching them effective coping strategies (Bristol et al., 1993; Holland & Holden, 2016).

Independent of the type of clinical approach that is applied, interveners should consider the psychological needs of the mothers and their children, and seek to fulfill these needs efficiently. While engaging in these clinical approaches, interveners should internalize and practice the essential skills, which are being sensitive, emphatic, non-judgmental, and supportive. In group psychotherapy, therapists also work as a part of a larger group providing the environment full of these skills. Feeling being listened to and supported in an emphatic and non-judgmental atmosphere, mothers and children feel free to open up themselves and talk about their inner feelings including shame, anger, guilt, and regret. Reliving the distress related to those emotions provides them new alternatives to build up a new kind of relationship both with themselves and their children.

Although previous research fairly widely documented the results of effectiveness studies targeting depressed mothers and their children, clinical studies which include mothers with various other psychological disorders are still an early stage. Given the chronicity and severity of symptoms, alongside the complexity of needs in mothers with psychological disorders, more research should be conducted targeting mothers with anxiety disorders, eating disorders, somatoform disorders, and schizophrenia, as well as with their children. The findings may suggest that the implementation of multi-level treatment approaches, which simultaneously focus on mother-child dyads' emerging needs may be essential. In addition to limited number of studies with mothers having various psychological disorders, fathers are usually not the targets of psychotherapy and intervention approaches. Although this chapter has focused on psychotherapy and intervention approaches, other programs may affect favorable outcomes, including massage therapy and group-based support. Furthermore, the preventive intervention starting up during pregnancy and maintaining after birth-giving may also be protective in preventing symptoms to become severe. More feasibility studies are needed to explore the techniques that clinical treatments use, to test whether parents perceive them as helpful, and to investigate their effectiveness in alleviating the symptom levels and relationship difficulties.

## REFERENCES


Abel, K. M., Webb, R., Salmon, M., Wan, M. W. & Appleby, L. (2005). The prevalence and predictors of parenting outcomes in a cohort of mothers with schizophrenia admitted for joint psychiatric care in England. *Journal of Clinical Psychiatry, 66*, 781–789.

Ainsworth, M. D. S., Blehar, M. C., Waters, E., & Wall, S. (1978). *Patterns of attachment: A psychological study of the strange situation.* Hillsdale, NJ: Erlbaum.

Armstrong, H. A., Wilks, C., & Melville, C. (2003). Clinical factors in group psychotherapy for parents of adolescents with disruptive behaviour disorders. *International Journal of Adolescent Medicine and Health, 15*, 21–30.

Bakermans-Kranenburg, M. J., van Ijzendoorn, M. H., & Juffer, F. (2003). Less is more: meta-analyses of sensitivity and attachment interventions in early childhood. *Psychological Bulletin, 129,* 195–215.

Bakermans-Kranenburg, M. J., van Ijzendoorn, M. H., & Juffer, F. (2005). Disorganized infant attachment and preventive interventions: a review and meta-analysis. *Infant Mental Health Journal, 26,* 191– 216.

Baradon, T., Broughton, C., Gibbs, I., James, J., Joyce, A., & Woodhead, J. (2005). *The practice of psychoanalytic parent–infant psychotherapy: Claiming the baby.* Hove, England: Routledge.

Barnes, D. L. (2006). Postpartum depression: Its impact on couples and marital satisfaction. *Journal of Systemic Therapies*, *25*, 25–42.

Blake, P. (2018). *Child and adolescent psychotherapy*. Routledge.

Bowlby, J. (1969/1982). *Attachment and loss: Vol. 1. Attachment.* New York: Basic Books, I.

Bristol, M. M., Gallagher, J. J., & Holt, K. D. (1993). Maternal depressive symptoms in autism: response to psychoeducational intervention. *Rehabilitation Psychology, 38*, 3–10.

Brown, G. W., & Moran, P. M. (1997). Single mothers, poverty and depression. *Psychological Medicine*, *27*, 21–33.

Burlingame, G. M., Fuhriman, A., & Johnson, J. E. (2001). Cohesion in group psychotherapy. *Psychotherapy: Theory, Research, Practice, Training, 38*, 373–379.

Cicchetti, D., & Toth, S. L. (1995). Developmental psychopathology and disorders of affect. In D. Cicchetti & D. Cohen (Eds.), *Developmental psychopathology, Vol. 2: Risk, disorder, and adaptation* (pp. 369–420). New York: Wiley.

Cicchetti, D., & Toth, S. L. (1998). The development of depression in children and adolescents. *American Psychologist, 53*, 221–241.

Cicchetti, D., Rogosch, F. A., & Toth, S. L. (2000). The efficacy of toddler-parent psychotherapy for fostering cognitive development in offspring of depressed mothers. *Journal of Abnormal Child Psychology*, *28*, 135–148.

Cicchetti, D., Rogosch, F. A., Toth, S. L. (2006). Fostering secure attachment in infants in maltreating families through preventive interventions. *Developmental Psychopathology, 18,* 623–649.

Cicchetti, D., Toth, S. L., & Rogosch, F. A. (1999). The efficacy of toddler-parent psychotherapy to increase attachment security in offspring of depressed mothers. *Attachment & Human Development*, *1*, 34–66.

Cooper, P. J., & Murray, L. (1997). Prediction, detection, and treatment of postnatal depression. *Archives of Disease in Childhood*, *77*, 97– 99.

Cramer, B. (1995). Short-term dynamic psychotherapy for infants and their parents. *Infant Psychiatry, 4*, 649–660.

Cuijpers, P., Weitz, E., Karyotaki, E., Garber, J., & Andersson, G. (2015). The effects of psychological treatment of maternal depression on children and parental functioning: a meta-analysis. *European Child and Adolescent Psychiatry*, 24, 237–245.

Dozier, M., & Roben, J. K. (2015). Attachment-related preventive interventions. In J. A. Simpson & S. W. Rholes (Eds.), *Attachment theory and research* (pp. 374–392). New York: Guilford Press.

Field, T., Pickens, J., Prodromidis, M., Malphurs, J., Fox, N., Bendell, D., Yando, R., Schanberg, S., & Kuhn, C. (2000). Targeting adolescent mothers with depressive symptoms for early intervention. *Adolescence, 35,* 382–414.

Fonagy, P., Sleed, M., & Baradon, T. (2016). Randomized controlled trial of parent–infant psychotherapy for parents with mental health problems and young infants. *Infant Mental Health Journal*, *37*, 97–114.

Frigerio, A., Porreca, A., Simonelli, A., & Nazzari, S. (2019). Emotional Availability in samples of mothers at high risk for depression and with substance use disorder. *Frontiers in Psychology*, *10*, 1–9.

Frost, K. (2012). The Ububele Baby Mat Project: A community-based parent-infant intervention at primary health care clinics in Alexandra Township, Johannesburg. *South African Journal of Psychology, 42*, 608–616.

Fukkink, R. G. (2008). Video feedback in widescreen: A meta-analysis of family programs. *Clinical Psychology Review*, *28*, 904–916.

Gopalan, G., Dean-Assael, K., Klingenstein, K., Chacko, A., & McKay, M. M. (2010). Caregiver depression and youth disruptive behavior difficulties. *Social Work in Mental Health*, *9*, 56–70.

Grote, N. K., Swartz, H. A., & Zuckoff, A. (2008). Enhancing interpersonal psychotherapy for mothers and expectant mothers on low incomes: Adaptations and additions. *Journal of Contemporary Psychotherapy*, *38*, 23–33.

Gruber, E. N., Kajević, M., Agius, M., & Martić-Biočina, S. (2006). Group psychotherapy for parents of patients with schizophrenia. *International Journal of Social Psychiatry*, *52*, 487–500.

Holland, G. W. O., & Holden, G. W. (2016). Changing orientations to corporal punishment: A randomized, control trial of the efficacy of a motivational approach to psycho-education. *Psychology of Violence, 6*, 233–242.

Hynd, S. & Khan, S. (2006). Video interaction guidance offered to mothers with postnatal depression: experiences from a pilot study. *Nordic Journal of Psychiatry, 60,* 234–238.

Ialongo, N. S., Rogosch, F. A., Cicchetti, D., Toth, S. L., Buckley, J., Petras, H., & Neiderhiser, J. (2006). A developmental psychopathology approach to the prevention of mental health disorders. In D. Cicchetti & D. J. Cohen (Eds.), *Developmental psychopathology: Theory and method* (p. 968–1018). John Wiley & Sons, Inc.

James, J. (2002). Developing a culture for change in group analytic psychotherapy for mothers and babies. *British Journal of Psychotherapy*, *19*, 77–91.

Juffer, F., Bakermans-Kranenburg, M. J., & Van IJzendoorn, M. (2017b). Pairing attachment theory and social learning theory in video-feedback intervention to promote positive parenting. *Current Opinion in Psychology, 15,* 189–194.

Juffer, F., Bakermans-Kranenburg, M. J., & Van IJzendoorn, M. H. (2017a). Video-feedback Intervention to promote Positive Parenting and Sensitive Discipline (VIPP-SD): Development and meta-analytical evidence of its effectiveness. In H. Steele & M. Steele (Eds.), *Handbook of attachment-based interventions* (pp. 1–26). Guilford Press.

Juffer, F., Bakermans-Kranenburg, M. J., & Van IJzendoorn, M. H. (2008b). *Manual VIPP-SD: Video-feedback program to promote positive parenting and sensitive discipline.* Netherlands: Leiden University.

Juffer, F., Bakermans-Kranenburg, M. J., & van Ijzendoorn, M. H. (2005). The importance of parenting in the development of disorganized attachment: evidence from a preventative intervention study in adoptive families. *Journal of Child Psychology Psychiatry, 46,* 263–274.

Kersting, A., Fisch, S., & Arolt, V. (2003). Outpatient psychotherapy for mothers–a new treatment. *Archives of Women's Mental Health, 6*, 65–69.

Kersting, A., Kuschel, S., Reutemann, M., Ohrmann, P., & Arolt, V. (2003). Outpatient psychotherapy for mothers—first empirical results. *Psychiatry: Interpersonal and Biological Processes*, *66*, 335–345.

Knoche, L. L., Edwards, C. P., Sheridan, S. M., Kupzyk, K. A., Marvin, C. A., Cline, K. D., & Clarke, B. L. (2012). Getting ready: Results of a randomized trial of a relationship-focused intervention on the parent–infant relationship in rural early head start. *Infant Mental Health Journal*, *33*, 439–458.

Kotwal, N., & Prabhakar, B. (2009). Problems faced by single mothers. *Journal of Social Sciences*, *21*, 197–204.

Koutra, K., Chatzi, L., Bagkeris, M., Vassilaki, M., Bitsios, P., & Kogevinas, M. (2013). Antenatal and postnatal maternal mental health as determinants of infant neurodevelopment at 18 months of age in a mother–child cohort (Rhea Study) in Crete, Greece. *Social Psychiatry and Psychiatric Epidemiology*, *48*, 1335–1345.

Licata, M., Zietlow, A. L., Träuble, B., Sodian, B., & Reck, C. (2016). Maternal emotional availability and its association with maternal psychopathology, attachment style insecurity and theory of mind. *Psychopathology*, *49*, 334–340.

Luster, T., & Okagaki, L. (2006). *Parenting: An ecological perspective* (Vol. 2). Routledge.

Luthar, S. S., & Suchman, N. E. (2000). Relational Psychotherapy Mothers' Group: A developmentally informed intervention for at- risk mothers. *Development and Psychopathology*, *12*, 235–253.

Marsack, C. N., & Samuel, P. S. (2017). Mediating effects of social support on quality of life for parents of adults with autism. *Journal of Autism and Developmental Disorders*, *47*, 2378–2389.

Mesman, G. R., Edge, N. A., McKelvey, L. M., Pemberton, J. L., & Holmes, K. J. (2017). Effects of maternal depression symptoms and alcohol use problems on child internalizing and externalizing behavior problems. *Journal of Child and Family Studies*, *26*, 2485–2494.

Murray, L., Cooper, P. J., Wilson, A., & Romaniuk, J. (2003). Controlled trial of the short- and long-term effect of psychological treatment of post-partum depression. *British Journal of Psychiatry, 182,* 420–427.

Nylen, K. J., Moran, T. E., Franklin, C. L., & O'hara, M. W. (2006). Maternal depression: A review of relevant treatment approaches for mothers and infants. *Infant Mental Health Journal: Official Publication of the World Association for Infant Mental Health*, *27*, 327–343.

Reich, S. M., Penner, E. K., Duncan, G. J., & Auger, A. (2012). Using baby books to change new mothers' attitudes about corporal punishment. *Child Abuse & Neglect, 36,* 108 –117.

Romans-Clarkson, S. E., Walton, V. A., Herbison, G. P., & Mullen, P. E. (1988). A study of women who refused to participate in a community survey of psychiatric disorder. *Australian & New Zealand Journal of Psychiatry*, *22*, 19–29.

Scholer, S. J., Hamilton, E. C., Johnson, M. C., & Scott, T. A. (2010). A brief intervention may affect parents' attitudes toward using less physical punishment. *Family & Community Health, 33,* 106–116.

Siegenthaler, E., Munder, T., & Egger, M. (2012). Effect of preventive interventions in mentally ill parents on the mental health of the offspring: systematic review and meta-analysis. *Journal of the American Academy of Child & Adolescent Psychiatry*, *51*, 8–17.

Smith, K. E., Landry, S. H., & Swank, P. R. (2005). The influence of decreased parental resources on the efficacy of a responsive parenting intervention. *Journal of Consulting and Clinical Psychology*, *73*, 711–720.

Stein, A., Woolley, H., Senior, R., Hertzmann, L., Lovel, M., Lee, J., Cooper, S., Wheatcroft, R., Challacombe, F., Patel, P., & Nicol-Harper, R. (2006). Treating disturbances in the relationship between mothers with bulimic eating disorders and their infants: a randomized, controlled trial of video feedback. *American Journal of Psychiatry, 163,* 899–906.

Sutton, A., & Hughes, L. (2005). The psychotherapy of parenthood: towards a formulation and valuation of concurrent work with parents. *Journal of Child Psychotherapy*, *31*, 169–188.

Swartz, H. A., Cyranowski, J. M., Cheng, Y., Zuckoff, A., Brent, D. A., Markowitz, J. C.,... & Frank, E. (2016). Brief psychotherapy for maternal depression: Impact on mothers and children. *Journal of the American Academy of Child & Adolescent Psychiatry*, *55*, 495–503.

Swartz, H. A., Frank, E., Zuckoff, A., et al. (2008). Brief interpersonal psychotherapy for depressed mothers whose children are receiving psychiatric treatment. *American Journal of Psychiatry*, 165, 1155–1162.

Tessier, R., Cristo, M., Velez, S., Giron, M., Figueroa de Calume, Z., & Ruiz Paláez, J. G. et al. (1998). Kangaroo mother care and the bonding hypothesis. *Pediatrics, 10,* 17–25.

Teti, D. M., Gelfand, D. M., Messinger, D. S., & Isabella, R. (1995). Maternal depression and the quality of early attachment: an examination of infants, preschoolers, and their mothers. *Developmental Psychology*, *31*, 364–376.

Tilley, S., & Chambers, M. (2000). An application of conjoint analysis to the process of psychiatric day hospital care. *Journal of Psychiatric Mental Health Nursing, 7*, 371–372.

Toth, S. L., Rogosch, F. A., Sturge-Apple, M., & Cicchetti, D. (2009). Maternal depression, children's attachment security, and representational development: An organizational perspective. *Child Development*, *80*, 192–208.

Van IJzendoorn, M. H., Juffer, F., & Duyvesteyn, M. G. C. (1995). Breaking the intergenerational cycle of insecure attachment: A review of the effects of attachment-based interventions on maternal sensitivity and infant security. *Journal of Child Psychology and Psychiatry, 36,* 225–248.

Wan, M. W., Moulton, S., & Abel, K. M. (2008). A review of mother–child relational interventions and their usefulness for mothers with schizophrenia. *Archives of Women's Mental Health*, *11*, 171– 179.

## BIOGRAPHICAL SKETCH

***Cansu Alsancak-Akbulut***

**Affiliation:** Ankara University

**Education:** PhD Candidate in Clinical Psychology

**Research and Professional Experience:** 2016 September – Present: Teaching Assistant in Ankara University

**Publications from the Last 3 Years:**

1) Alsancak-Akbulut, C., Sarıtaş-Atalar, D., & Metin-Orta, İ. (2020). Effective parenting within an integrative framework of emotional availability and domains-of-socialization. In *Family Conflict: Perspectives, Management and Outcomes*. Nova Publishing.
2) Alsancak-Akbulut, C., Sahin Acar, B., & Sumer, N. (2020). Effect of video-feedback intervention on Turkish mothers' sensitivity and physical intrusiveness: a randomized control trial. *Attachment & Human Development*, 1-19.
3) Sümer, N., Metin-Orta, İ., Alsancak-Akbulut, C., Salman-Engin, S., İlden-Koçkar, A., Şahin-Acar, B., Akkol-Solakoğlu, S., Aran, Ö., Işılay, D. S., Kavaklı, B., Memişoğlu-Şanlı, A., Sağel-Çetiner, E., Türe, D., Üstünel A. Ö., & Yaşar, B. (2020). The effects of video-feedback intervention to promote positive parenting-

sensitive discipline for maternal sensitivity in Turkey. *Journal of Turkish Psychology, 35*(85), 1-17.

4) Şahin-Acar, B., Bahtiyar-Saygan, B., Alsancak-Akbulut, C., & Sağel-Çetiner, E. (2019). Reunion after a long day: Mother-child dyads' unshared memory conversations. *Cognitive Development, 52*, 100822.

In: Psychotherapy
Editor: Hayley Boyd

ISBN: 978-1-53618-877-6


*Chapter 10*

# IT'S A POLITICAL AGE: THE CURRENT AGE, SUBJECTIVITY AND PSYCHOTHERAPY

***Nissim Avissar****

Kibbutzim College of Education, Tel-Aviv, Israel

## ABSTRACT

This article deals with the era in which we live, an era marked by rapid change on a multitude of planes. The Corona virus pandemic has accelerated and exaggerated the existing trend. The present time is characterized by volatility, uncertainty, complexity and ambiguity (VUCA). These sharp changes necessarily shape or re-construct human subjectivity in ways that bring about further changes both in the individual experience and needs, in interpersonal relations and in social and political trends. In view of these changes, I believe it to be very apposite to revisit psychotherapy: its theories, tools and activities. I would like to argue that politically sensitive or socially responsible approaches, that will be described briefly, are bound to play a major role in the renewal of psychotherapy. They may have a unique contribution to the effort of psychotherapists to reconnect to the communities and societies in which they operate, and to become agents of social change.

---

* Corresponding Author's E-mail: Email: nissimav@gmail.com.

**Keywords:** culture, context, postmodernity, psychotherapy, social-responsibility, subjectivity, VUCA

## INTRODUCTION

> All of us are, willy-nilly, by design or by default, on the move. We are on the move even if, physically, we stay put: immobility is not a realistic option in a world of permanent change (Bauman, 1998, p. 2).

We live in exceptional times. It is an era characterized by sharp shifts and turns, whose dimensions and consequences it is too early to oversee. The last decades have seen the removal of constraints and the overthrow of rules which defined human existence, it would seem, forever. This was made possible as a result of technological developments and global-political processes. Traditional sources of security and stability, as a result, became extremely compromised. A person's connection to a place and a community; the social structure and familiar frameworks which had been so self-evident – the known rules of the game according to which life is lived – these were all pillars of a stable life for most of humanity, yet they held those who lived in the margins in isolation and suffering. Now, possibilities present themselves: individuals who live in the margins and all kinds of minority groups stand a greater chance of finding solidarity and support, to build a community (whether or not virtual) and to gain legitimacy and social acceptance. Those, by contrast, who learned to rely on the familiar rules are bound to feel the ground shifting under their feet. And so, needs and afflictions change too. The Corona virus pandemic has once again disrupted the prior global-cultural trend. At present time, it is too early to consider the repercussions of this major event.

In this article I reflect on the era in which we live, an era marked by rapid change on a multitude of planes. In view of these changes, I believe it to be very apposite to revisit psychotherapy: its tools and activities. I would like to argue that professional-political approaches like the ones described in this article are bound to play a major role in the renewal of psychotherapy.

## Subjectivity

As Jacques Derrida (1982) showed us, the concept of a subject and hence of subjectivity, is a complex one. On the one hand, being a subject means agency and the capacity to construct and interpret reality. Therefore, subjectivity entails individual choice and responsibility. This is why this concept is so closely linked to western thought following the seventeenth century and more specifically to the enlightenment movement: "it grounds the possibility of freedom – freedom from determination and domination, freedom to be self-determining and sovereign" (Flax, 1993, p. 92).

But at the same time, Derrida argues, a condition to becoming a subject is being subjected to language, society, and norms. From this perspective, the concept of subjectivity encompasses the complex interrelations between individual and society. Hadar (2013) articulates the same idea differently. Referring to the work of Lacan, Levinas, Jessica Benjamin and others, he claims that one needs the other's subjectivity to become a subject (i.e., to develop her or his own subjectivity). Hadar writes: "the *other* takes a formative role in the constitution of the subject and the ethics of being a subject" (p. 211). The other may well be society, culture, or politics and not necessarily a personal other. Hadar goes on to draw insights from this idea in regard to psychotherapeutic processes and to social involvement. Hollander (2006) refers to citizens' and psychotherapists' social responsibility "to understand the complex nature of subjectivity as it is formed in relation to a sociosymbolic order composed of asymmetrical relations of power and force" (p. 164).

Along the same lines, Emerson and Frosh (2009) write about "the *psychosocial* subject" and link their interest in it to critical narrative analysis. Here too we may find similar complexity, as the critical perspective focuses on the potential impact of context - and more specifically on the power relations in that context - on the lives (and subjectivity) of individuals. Simultaneously, the narrative perspective emphasizes the value of unique voices and individual life stories and their potential impact on society. This means that both society and individuals have power and responsibility. Indeed, society and its individual members entertain a relationship which, while not symmetrical, is certainly mutual.

Thus, self and other, individual and society, subjectivity and political reality are intertwined. Their relationship is marked by a dialectical tension within the concept of subjectivity which one must hold to avoid over-simplification, determinism (responsibility lies with society only), or blaming the victim (responsibility lies exclusively with the individual). Let us now examine some uniquely contemporary features of subjectivity.

## LIQUID SUBJECTIVITY?

Zygmunt Bauman (2000), the sociologist, uses the term “liquid modernity” to describe the present time with its typical mobility and constant transformation. Both underline the characteristic time/space relations marking this historical period. Bauman draws a connection between the dimension of time on one hand, and consumer society and “instant” culture on the other. Disposable products are made to supply instant satisfaction to subjects whose consciousness moves fast in constant search of the next stimulation. Attention is directed outward and flashes – it goes after a new excitement, finds it, loses interest, and moves on. Satisfaction has to be immediate in order to allow the consumerist search for happiness to go on. The optimal duration is the shortest possible for the act of consumption. One can say, in a sense, that this is an addictive and shallow consciousness which has grown dependent on consumption articles and increasingly intense stimuli in order to achieve a sense of calm and meaningfulness. Such conditions produce an “empty self” (Cushman, 1990) and psychological poverty (Wachtel, 1989) which in turn generate a constant sense of lack. The spatial dimension involves the ever-increasing effortlessness of changing location and the lessening constraints on movement in space (whether geographical or virtual). More people are on the move, whether temporarily (as tourists) or on a more fixed basis (as migrants). Others are in motion more steadily, leading what amounts to a nomadic existence. Traditional borders are disappearing: new worlds are being discovered, and if we don't discover them ourselves, then they somehow find us out. The texture of society, as a result, changes into something more heterogeneous and old norms become obsolete. As with other aspects of the current era, this involves a change that could on the one hand open possibilities and enlarge potential freedoms or to destabilize things and sow horror, on the other. Bauman writes: "Thrown into a vast open sea with no navigation charts and all the marker buoys sunk and barely visible, we have only two choices left: we may rejoice in the breath-taking vistas of new discoveries - or we may tremble out of fear of drowning" (1998, p. 85).

The liquid character of the times, the fast motion in space and time, all of these obviously leave their imprint on the structure of our identity. Bauman writes:

> That work of art which we want to mould out of the friable stuff of life is called 'identity'. Whenever we speak of identity, there is at the back of our minds a faint image of harmony, logic, consistency: all those things which the flow of our experience seems - to our perpetual despair - so grossly and abominably to lack. The search for identity is the ongoing struggle to arrest or slow down the flow, to solidify the fluid, to give form to the formless (2000, p. 82).

These are, in other words, times marked by a crisis of identity; times when even the inner pegs that supply the sense of continuity and stability of self experience have lost hold in a soil that has grown shifty and precarious. Identity too – just like disposable consumer articles or our endless zapping between TV stations in search of meaning and interest – identity too has become liquid.

Having served as a stable ground for identity, the family too is now undergoing an upheaval. Changes in the structure of the family and the variety of new types that have joined the traditional ones (one parent, single sex parents, parents who live separately, and so on) crucially affect the individual who grows up in them. Affected, also, are attitudes to authority, to its institutions and to society at large (Salecl, 2000). The rejection of authority, however, does not only liberate: it also sparks the subject's anger and disappointment with authority for having betrayed her or him. This global-personal process has found expression in a number of current anti-social phenomena which are easily observable, both in society at large and in the clinic. Beny Mor (1999) calls the self experience in the current era "the suffocated self" – a self that thirsts after intimate contact and suffers from a sense of "disconnection and emptiness" as well as "splitting, alienation and loneliness"; he writes:

> Attachment theories make a point of the importance of secure primary attachment, which then forms the basis for interpersonal openness in the future and the ability for emotional self-regulation [...] The social atmosphere and our modes of existence get in the way of creating experiences that provide the sense of holding, security, continuity and belonging needed to realize internal freedom and authentic identity (p. 23).

When this is the state of affairs, it is no wonder that the individual cries out in diverse ways and forms which is clearly audible through the silence of all the 'suffocated selves' who are unable to raise their voices.

Is this a process that consists mainly of the extension of the field of possibilities, or rather an enforced development that limits individuals' capacity for happiness? As said, while for some people this cultural change opens new possibilities, it silences others, removing the ground that held them. According to Bauman (1998) there is a logic to who gains from this and who has lost: it is essentially a class-based division that discriminates between people with means and those who have poor resources.

The elites' link-up with the global world means mobility and evasiveness. It is fairly simple for the latter to maneuver between these two modes of life – the local and the global – using the one wherever there's a problem with the other. They move about in an ex-territorial domain which has many laws but none of them binding. This results in an intolerable anomaly wherever it concerns the attitude towards members of different classes on the part of those who have authority and the law on their side. For Bauman, the consequence is "the identification of crime with the (always local) 'underclass' – or, which amounts to much the same, the criminalization of poverty" (p. 125). As a result of this injustice, disadvantaged individuals and groups are pushed into the margins of society, depriving them of the right to reap the benefits of the present era, its plethora of possibilities.

This being the case, frustration piles up and this may lead to explosive, angry situations, whether on the individual or the collective levels. Among the numerous varied occurrences that represent the change in social power structures are events such as the UK vote to leave the EU (Brexit), and the election of Donald Trump as president of the United States. Worldwide political phenomena like Al-Qaeda or ISIS may also be viewed and understood within such framework. It is not hard to see the connection between these processes and the social and political uprisings such as the Arab spring and social protests (e.g., in Wall Street, Tunisia, Tel-Aviv and other places). There's an outcry for a new order, a different, more equal division of power. The fact that this experience is simultaneously extremely personal and collective is what makes it so powerful. Individuals who live at great distances from one another, share personal experiences that, today, they can communicate via the social networks and by other means. This enables the creation of a strong community. This social dynamism can be likened to the movement of a wave that gathers strength and then floods the sands, the existing reality. And so we return to the tension between an old, solid modernity and its present, liquid version.

## Psychotherapy in Context

These processes of change demand a re-examination of the objectives and methods of psychotherapy. Right now, it is hard to predict how the above described social changes will affect psychotherapy. Still, one channel may include fundamental change in the way psychotherapeutic conceptions and tools relate to the individual's everyday reality, and the annulment of the sharp distinction between the internal and the external worlds. The current cultural revolution, in other words, is bound to lead to the renewed inclusion of politics in the therapeutic discourse and to a focusing on the political aspects of both personal and professional experience so that they make come to be a renewed anchor for liquid identity. As mentioned, politics which represents power relations, assumes the existence of asymmetric relations which impact both identity and well-being. Once we recognize the political nature of identity, as well as thc political nature of psychotherapy, a complex examination becomes possible of the interrelations that contributed to the formation of identity in the past and to the constitution of perceptions (of self and the of the world) in the present. Omitting either one side in this equation is likely to result in damage or suffering, either due to the individual's guilt (internal focus) or by turning her or him into a victim (external focus). The political (cultural, social) third may well help us extricate ourselves from this binary model so as to enable an inclusive view of the individual in his or her changing context. I believe that we are at the height of a paradigm revolution and as is the case with every revolution, there will be those who will suffer as a result. But we cannot freeze and not move on. Such stasis, indeed, would be damaging. As Samuels (2006) writes:

> Foreclosure on politics, the privileging and valorizing of the internal over the external, may, as we stagger through the first decade of the new century, itself constitute a bad clinical practice. From today's perspective, maybe I do want or need to some bad practice as I change my practice. Those who do not or cannot change their practices may, from tomorrow's point of view, be ones guilty of bad practice (p. 16).

Any initial attempts, including the present one, to incorporate politics into therapeutic discourse and practices can only be expected to be hesitant and somewhat clumsy. That's the 'bad practice' which may lead to better work, practices better adjusted to the mood and needs of the here and now.

Psychotherapy, facing contemporary challenges, can take on a more significant social or political role. It can assume the role of the flag-bearer of an ethics which may support every person's right to live well in conditions of basic security – both physical and mental. If this is what they want to achieve, psychotherapeutic communities will have to clarify and redefine their values – to clarify what kind of relations they want to entertain with political domains. They will have to consider what types of power are at play in the reality in which they operate (including those powers that affect and shape them), and to situate themselves in this field while keeping constant track of their own actions and their effects. Psychotherapy will gain status and have effective power only when its messages – explicit and implicit; theoretical and practical – show consistency, integrity and sincerity. If one takes a clear and uncompromising position this also requires dealing with the disagreement of, and conflict with, those who subscribe to a clashing approach. This may well lead to real struggle and criticism, from within and without. In my opinion, this is a necessary condition for change.

## Politically Sensitive and Socially Responsible Psychotherapy

Seeing a person in the social-cultural context and spotlighting external-reality-related causes of suffering (alongside the individual's own responsibility) constitutes both a choice of perspective and a form of action, political and therapeutic. For when the bond between a person and her or his environment is strengthened this is likely to underwrite their sense of belonging and solidarity, stimulate community building and the development of social support networks. All this is in sharp contrast with the individualism and interpersonal alienation unwittingly encouraged by traditional intra-psychic models. Indeed, rather than a perspective that assumes a person's source of suffering is intrinsic to themselves, which then leads to a life story that is tantamount to a narrative of aberration and failure (and in fact puts the client in the role of the victim), recognition of the social and cultural factors in personal suffering is likely to assist in processes of re-framing of the events – from a narrative of victimhood and helplessness to one of overcoming and determination. A position that makes room for social-political context, moreover, will help the client evolve a sense of the external factors of his or her suffering. This will reduce feelings of failure and guilt and encourage a pro-active attitude. An opening for initiative and action in external reality will thus come about (for both therapist and client, together and each separately), with the objective to introduce change. While these things are bound to make a significant social contribution to the community, they also offer a source of personal satisfaction and self-worth deriving from the act of giving and from feeling that one manages to live a meaningful life in an oppressive reality. In the current cultural context, marked as it is by the breakdown of traditional sources of security and stability along with an exponential growth in channels of information which threaten to flood us – therapists and clients alike are bound to develop a sense of self-adequacy and control and to evolve a type of internal anchor that will help them cope in a world they experience as chaotic. Still it must be noted that these are not universally valid principles. Their dogmatic deployment can even affect some therapists adversely, as is always likely where there is an absence of judgment and critical thinking. Sometimes, obviously, it will be through a focus on pathological elements or through a process of soul searching that keeps the outside advisedly out that the client is best empowered. I am nevertheless convinced that in our times a politically conscious approach which includes the individual's social-cultural context is both valuable and preferable.

This emphasis on context is one of five principles presented in the earlier mentioned empowerment model of McWirther and McWirther (2007). Though these authors focus their attention on clinical training and supervision, I believe their model can be adjusted to politically sensitive psychotherapy. So, McWirther and McWirther describe five principles: collaboration, context, critical consciousness, competence, and community. I will consider each of these briefly.

- Collaboration – refers to the "joint definitions of the problems to be addressed, goals of counseling, and possible interventions and strategies for change and growth" (p.420). This actually also includes transparency and partnership, which imply renunciation of power. Collaboration, here, does not refer to its more common meaning: the client's submissive response to the therapist, but rather clients' vital involvement in any decision making. In the absence of such collaboration, "the counselor risks reinforcing passivity and neediness in the client, misunderstanding the nature and meaning of the client's difficulties, and developing interventions that are inconsistent with the client's values, culture, ideology, goals, and skills" (ibid.).
- Context – over and beyond what was already mentioned, this means understanding clients' and therapists' life by familiarizing oneself with their family and community environment, their socio-political history, their socio-economic status, their culture and values. This amounts to a detailed and realistic clarification of the client's life situation: the conditions in which his or her personality evolves and can be made sense of.
- Critical Consciousness – relates to "individuals' ability to examine themselves within their life contexts, and to see themselves as actors in those contexts rather than merely as individuals who are acted on" (p.423). This component, therefore, includes dimensions of awareness and action and requires commitment to an ongoing examination of contexts and their mutual interactions, especially on the part of the therapist.
- Competence – which refers to this approach's key emphasis on clients' competence and skills throughout the therapeutic process. If a therapy that pivots on weaknesses and hardships leads to their

entrenchment and even further amplification, then a focus on clients' strengths may bring about their empowerment. What might appear as a neutral description in fact represents the result of selective attention which constitutes a choice that is formative of reality. It happens that our own preferred position as therapists gets in the way of perceiving and getting ourselves acquainted with clients' own subjective perception and interpretation of reality. Shifting our own perspective as therapists, we may recognize additional resources and competences (either existing or potential) available to our clients. Ignoring these will support processes of disempowerment, while the concerted effort to find and focus on them will allow the client to recognize them him or herself, thus adding to their sense of self-effectiveness and self-worth.

- Community – this might be the component that is most conspicuously absent from conventional therapeutic discourse. Community relates to the possibility of promoting through therapy individuals' identification with and involvement in the community. It is achieved by the clarification of a person's sense of belonging, the quality of his or her relationships, etc. Community may be defined by means of ethnic, religious or extended familial connections, as a shared way of living or as a group of friends and or of other relations. The link to community supports identity consolidation by means of an awareness of the past. And equally it acts as a source of hope and strength, support and challenge, relationship and contribution. This latter factor, being able to contribute to other people, offers an opportunity to connect to others and collaborate with them, as well as being a source of self-worth. Elizabeth Vera and Suzette Speight (2007) present a long list of functions which a socially involved therapist may assume in the attempt to promote social justice. They choose to focus on three practical interventions: advocacy, outreach, and prevention. All of these can be deployed in individual forms of therapy and are likely to help in advancing clients as well as the community in which they live.

- Advocacy – is a type of therapeutic intervention aimed to enhance the realization of clients' rights when these are either denied or likely to be denied. In this case clients are concretely represented at institutional bodies, authorities, and so on, with the aim of challenging the inherent injustice of a certain policy (including for instance its bureaucratic rules) or to remove it entirely. This encompasses a wide range of possible activities, from making a phone call on behalf of clients all the way to taking legal steps to ensure their rights are being respected. This is a tool of social action in the service of empowering disadvantaged individuals and groups. Such action may take one of three forms: support for clients in representing themselves more efficiently; direct representation at institutions or vis a vis policy makers or indirect representation by means of training professionals who work with deprived populations.
- Outreach – though this is a better known notion, it is actually hardly practiced among therapists. Outreach requires therapists to leave their work surroundings and enter that of their clients or potential clients. Such venturing outside the familiar boundaries of the clinic and into the social reality is likely to expand therapists' knowledge about clients and their specific surroundings. It conveys a message to the effect that therapists are willing to take risks and initiatives and indicates their openness towards society in general and those who find themselves in its margins. Outreach, too, can take several forms: as part of a traditional therapeutic framework (house calls) or through a planned approach of those who for a variety of reasons (cultural, economic, geographical or otherwise) are unable to get to a place where assistance is offered.
- Prevention – proactivity is not a novel notion in psychology. Yet, as Vera and Speight comment, research shows that therapists don't consider it central to their work. Preventive action is likely to be especially effective with disadvantaged social groups that live in an environment marked by stress factors, often of the type involving prejudice, racism, or oppression. Problems like

> substance abuse, violence, high school dropout rates and unemployment are frequent in poor communities or communities of cultural or ethnic minorities. Such populations, however, also have limited access to relevant knowledge about mental health, nor is there much early prevention activity. One advantage of prevention activity is that it is relatively easy to incorporate in existing support structures of the mental health services, including structures for individual therapy. All this type of action requires is awareness and relevant training.

Some further concrete tools to promote therapists' involvement in the community and in politics are added by Kayla Weiner (1991). Practical suggestions like this may not suit every therapeutic environment but they illustrate a mode of political-therapeutic thinking and consciousness. The author argues that everything in the clinic constitutes a personal-political statement. Every component or feature of the clinic can be interpreted accordingly – including its size and the objects in it. All of these (as well as whatever is *not* in the clinic) amount to a message in relation to which the therapeutic discourse is conducted. Even though this is always the case, only few therapists will make use of this fact for therapeutic purposes. When the therapeutic objective includes a clearer political statement, a degree of courage is also required. In this regard, Weiner argues: "fear of being visible and therefore in possible danger, and the fear of being singled out by others as 'not nice', often keeps people from taking actions that they would otherwise like to take. It is therefore important for the therapist to be proactive and intentional in being a role model for her/his clients" (p.119). Awareness and involvement are already noticeable in the smallest details of the therapeutic environment. Thus, Weiner suggests to put up an announcement board in the waiting area because it can serve a variety of therapy-related purposes. Information that has some common interest may be shared in this way; the notice board may for instance display how various people are involved in the community, present a range of perspectives and ideas, or raise consciousness on some issue. If there are magazines in the waiting area, their nature, obviously, carries therapeutic significance testifying, among other things, to how the therapist perceives her or his clients. Another example is the following: if there is a water dispenser in the clinic the therapist may choose not to supply disposable cups and rather ask clients to bring their own cup or, alternatively, to rinse the non-disposable one they used. This type of action may encourage conversation about environmental issues, raise consciousness of possible damage, and suggest non-polluting solutions as well as action for a clean environment. To conclude, Weiner writes: "by assisting clients to realize that there are small things we can control in our environment, we can lead them to realize there are larger things over which they have control" (p.118).

The above tools illustrate modes of making socially responsible or politically sensitive therapy work. They are merely illustrations because the range of possible actions this position entails is endless. This type of therapy is likely to include individually–based interventions, even of the kind that is in consonance with conventional therapeutic approaches, along with interventions on the community and social levels. But we are dealing with a general rationale for understanding people and their development in terms of their interaction with social-political forces, a rationale which yields therapeutic insights, rather than with a method. In my view, in fact, any effort to formulate an explicit method for politically sensitive therapeutic work would be a contradiction in terms because the key notion 'political' is elusive and subversive, requiring specifically calibrated judgment each and every time. Still, a rationale can be feasibly formulated as well as tools for effective work in complex life situations.

## CONCLUSION

For a long time politics was considered off limits by mainstream psychotherapy. So, generations of therapists were instructed to keep away from any visible public activity, especially those that might give away their political affinities. Such avoidance, however, of direct involvement in politics in the narrow sense is only a small aspect of a much wider ranging phenomenon. Even in therapeutic practice and theory very little attention was devoted to how broad political factors (such as ethnicity, gender, or class) affect mental well-being and to how to refer to any social and political issues that might emerge in the course of therapy. Today, I believe, professional-psychotherapeutic communities are seeking a way back to the societies in which they operate, after years of detachment resulting in distrust and alienation. This process requires a professional change of mindset. I believe that the professional view that may serve individuals and groups in the present age is one that encompasses both individuals and contexts – cultural, social and political. From here it's a short way to include principles and methods like the ones discussed earlier in the everyday professional practice. That means, practicing a politically sensitive and socially responsible psychotherapy that espiers to promote social justice and well-being for all human beings (i.e., not only clients). This conscious and critical mode of work may enable the professional discourse and practice to transform themselves in ways that concord the wide cultural and political changes that affect subjectivity and human needs. A psychology that closes itself to the world in which it operates and that doesn't engage in a constant dynamic of self-examination, will end up as a tool of oppression. Such practice is irrelevant in this day and age is doomed to become obsolete.

## References

Bauman Z. (1998). *Globalization: The Human Consequence*. New York, NY: Columbia University Press.

Bauman Z. (2000). *Liquid Modernity*. Cambridge: Polity Press.

Cushman P. (1990). Why the Self is Empty: Toward a Historically Situated Psychology. *American psychologist*, 45 (5), 599-611.

Derrida J. (1982). Différance (translated by Alan Bass). In *Margins of Philosophy* (pp. 3-27). Chicago: University of Chicago Press.

Emerson P. and Frosh S. (2009). *Critical Narrative Analysis in Psychology: A guide to Practice* (Revised Edition), New York, NY: Palgrave-Macmillan.

Flax J. (1993). *Disputed Subjects: Essays on psychoanalysis, Politics and Philosophy*, New York, NY: Routledge.

Hadar U. (2013). *Psychoanalysis and Social Involvement: Interpretation and Action,* New York, NY: Palgrave-Macmillan.

Hollander N. C. (2006), Psychoanalysis and the Problem of Bystander in Times of Terror. In: Layton L., Hollander N. C. and Gutwill S. (Eds.), *Psychoanalysis, Class and Politics: Encounters in the Clinical Setting*, New York, NY: Routledge, pp. 154-165.

McWhirter E. H. and McWhirter B. T. (2007). Grounding Clinical Training and Supervision in an Empowerment Model. In, Aldarondo E. (Ed.), *Advancing Social Justice through Clinical Practice* (pp. 417-442). Lawrence Erlbaum Associates.

Mor B. (1999). 'Suffocated Self' – Postmodern cultural Influences on the Individual Psyche. *Sihot: Israel Journal of Psychotherapy*, 14 (1), 20-27 [Hebrew].

Samuels A. (2006). Working Directly with Political, Social, and Cultural Material in the Therapy Session. In: Layton L., Hollander N. C. and Gutwill S. (Eds.), *Psychoanalysis, Class and Politics: Encounters in the Clinical Setting*. New York, NY: Routledge, pp. 11-28.

Salecl R. (2000). *(Per)versions of love and hate*. London: Verso.

Vera E. M. and Speight S. L. (2007), "Advocacy, Outreach, and Prevention: Integrating Social Action Roles in Professional Training", in: Aldarondo E. (Ed.), *Advancing Social Justice through Clinical Practice* (pp. 373-390). Lawrence Erlbaum Associates.

Weiner K. M. (1988). "Methods of Incorporating Political/Social Action into the Therapy Session", in: Hill M. (Ed.), *Feminist Therapy as a Political Act* (pp. 113-123). Binghampton, NY: Harrington park press.

Whachtel P. L. (1989). *The Poverty of Affluence: A Psychological Portrait of the American Way of Life*, New York, NY: Free Press.

# INDEX

## A



## B

## C

## D



## E

## F



## G



## H

## I



## L



## M

## Q

## R



## S

## T

## V



## W